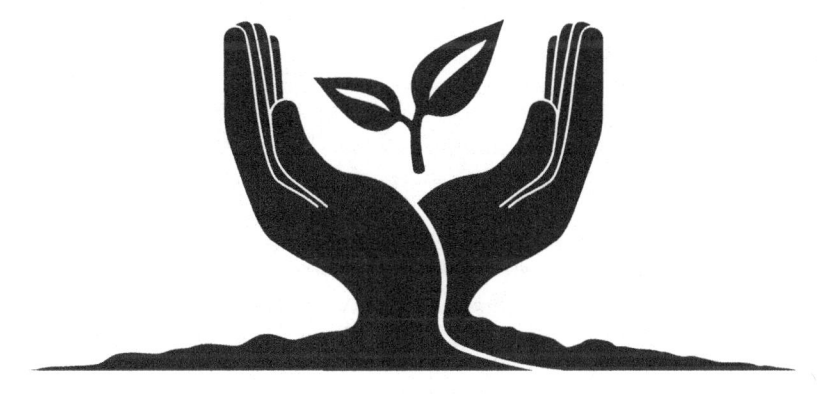

ROOTS OF POSITIVE CHANGE
Optimizing Health Care with Positive Psychology

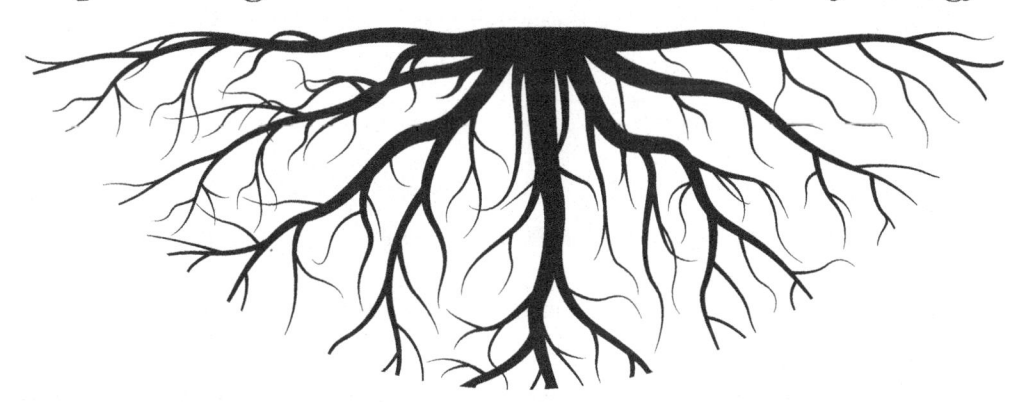

© 2019 American College of Lifestyle Medicine. All rights reserved. Printed in the United States.
American College of Lifestyle Medicine
PO Box 6432
Chesterfield, MO 63006
Published in collaboration with ©HealthType LLC

No part of this book may be reproduced, stored in a retrieval system or transmitted, in any form or by and means, electronic, mechanical, photocopying, recording, or otherwise, without the prior permission of the American College of Lifestyle Medicine.
Roots of Positive Change: Optimizing Health Care with Positive Psychology (BKR784-6A)

ISBN: 978-0-9888631-1-8
Book layout and cover design: Becky Hansen
HealthType LLC
PO Box 1461
Fair Oaks, CA 95628

Dr. Lianov's dedication and leadership in promoting collaboration across the fields of lifestyle medicine, positive psychology, and health care innovation puts her at the forefront of a new era of health care for advancing total well-being. This handbook, not only makes the case for positive psychology as an important new pillar of a healthy lifestyle, but also tackles early steps to redesign care to make this approach feasible for the medical setting. This is a must-read for health care practitioners who want to make a major difference in their practices, academic and professional communities and personal lives.

Jill Waalen, MD, MS, MPH, FACPM
Senior Scientist, Digital Medicine
Scripps Research Translational Institute

As a lifestyle medicine physician and educator, I consider the mindbody relationship foundational to successful behavior modification and holistic health of patients and providers alike. Evidence and experience show us compellingly that the field of positive psychology is instrumental in effectively leveraging this relationship, and I am thrilled by the arrival of this significant and pioneering endeavor! The authors thoughtfully champion the emerging movement of positive psychology in medical care. They inspire us to apply these strategies to established healthcare systems. Useful, practical tips for behavior coaching, treatment prescriptions, health team engagement, patient interactions, quality improvement processes, and practitioner well-being, make the field of positive psychology come to life vividly for the medical professional.

Kaylan A. Baban, MD, MPH, Chief Wellness Officer
Director, Lifestyle Medicine Program School of Medicine & Health Sciences
George Washington University

Integrating lifestyle medicine and positive psychology into clinical care has the potential to improve patient outcomes and reduce burnout of clinical professionals. This book, the first of its kind, reviews the underlying scientific framework, describes examples of successful interventions using these approaches, and outlines strategies to integrate these concepts into healing environments. Authored by leaders in medicine and psychology, it has the potential to spark an evolution in the practice of medicine.

Michael P. O'Donnell, MBA, MPH, PhD
CEO, Art and Science of Health Promotion Institute
Editor in Chief Emeritus, American Journal of Health Promotion

Dedication

This book is dedicated to all physicians, health professionals, health professionals-in-training, students, researchers, patients, parents, and families. We share the common driver in life to be happy and healthy and to thrive. We want to feel well in order to pursue our individual and common goals and experience life to the fullest. Our humanity draws us together. The ideas in this book offer hopeful approaches that may uplift us to achieve these goals…and to answer our "why."

Roots of Positive Change
Optimizing Health Care with Positive Psychology

Table of Contents

About ACLM 2
Acknowledgements 3
Foreword (Barbara Fredrickson) 5
Preface 7
Chapter 1: The Evolution of Two Interdependent Fields: Lifestyle Medicine and Positive Psychology 9
Chapter 2: Healthy Lifestyle Practices and Emotional Well-Being: A Reciprocal Relationship 19
Chapter 3: Positive Psychology Interventions 31
Chapter 4: Designing Health Care Practice to Harness Positive Psychology 43
Chapter 5: Bringing the Positive Psychology Approach to the Exam Room 55
Chapter 6: Harnessing Positive Psychology Techniques in Health Behavior Change Coaching 63
Chapter 7: Personalizing Positive Psychology Interventions 75
Chapter 8: Quality Improvement of Positive Psychology Strategies in Health Care ... 85
Chapter 9: Physician and Health Professional Well-Being Based in Positive Psychology 97
Chapter 10: Positive Psychology in Medical Education and Beyond: Teaching, Modeling, Integrating, and Advocating 111
Chapter 11: Positive Psychology Research in Health Care 121
Chapter 12: Positive Psychology Resources 129
Epilogue: Planning the Way Forward 145
Appendix A: PERMA Model 149
Appendix B: Key Positive Psychology Intervention Studies 151
Appendix C: Emotional Well-Being Assessment Tools 157
Appendix D: Self-Rating Strengths 163
Appendix E: Personality Self-Assessment to Guide Selecting Positive Psychology Interventions 165
Appendix F: Sample Positive Psychology Curriculum 173
About the Editor 177
About the Authors 179

AMERICAN COLLEGE OF
Lifestyle Medicine

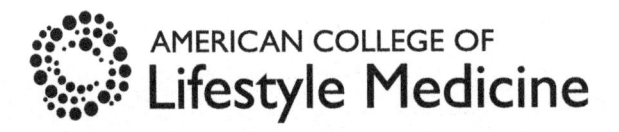

About ACLM

Vision:
A world in which physicians and allied health professionals
have been trained and certified in evidence-based lifestyle medicine,
integrating healthful behaviors into their own lives,
while incorporating a lifestyle medicine-first approach to treating root
causes of lifestyle-related diseases into their clinical practices.

American College of Lifestyle Medicine

The American College of Lifestyle Medicine (ACLM) is the medical professional association for those dedicated to the advancement and clinical practice of lifestyle medicine as the foundation of a transformed and sustainable system of health care delivery. More than a professional association, ACLM is a galvanized force for change. ACLM addresses the need for quality education and certification, supporting its members in their individual practices and their collective mission to domestically and globally promote lifestyle medicine as the first treatment option, as opposed to a first option of treating symptoms and consequences with expensive, ever-increasing qualities of pills and procedures. ACLM members are united in their desire to identify and eradicate the cause of disease, striving for sustainable health, sustainable health care and a sustainable world–as all are inextricably connected. For more information, visit www.lifestylemedicine.org. For information about certification in the field of lifestyle medicine, please visit www.ablm.co.

Acknowledgements

I'd like to express sincere gratitude to the individuals whose support was invaluable in producing this book.

A tremendous thank you is owed to Susan Benigas for her ongoing leadership at the American College of Lifestyle Medicine (ACLM). Her support to promote total well-being and to advocate for positive psychology as a key element of lifestyle medicine and health care in general provides an essential "home" for this work.

Members of the ACLM Happiness Science and Positive Health Committee (some of whom authored chapters of this book) have also been great leaders in promoting positive psychology in health care and have supported the need for the type of practitioner guidance offered in this book: Grace Caroline Barron, Kristen Collins, Ingrid Edshteyn, Janani Krishnaswami, Rachel Millstein, Joe Raphael, and Anne Wallace (co-authors); and Paresh Jaini, Jenny Lee, Noémie Le Pertel, Kathi Norman, Sondra Redmont, and Deepa Sannidhi.

George Guthrie and David Ferriss, who have been advocates on the topic of positive psychology and health, reviewed and provided insights that helped enrich the content. Anne Wallace served, not only as an author of two chapters, but also reviewed and edited the entire manuscript. Samantha Gallion, copy editor, and Becky Hansen, who designed the book cover and developed the formatting, were instrumental in the final product.

Thank you all!
– Liana Lianov

Foreward

Making Positive Change: A New Age of Positive Psychology and Health

Research in the field of positive psychology has expanded in numerous directions over the past three decades. One of the most exciting and potentially impactful areas of this research examines the effect of positive psychology activities, not only on subjective well-being, but also on physical health. My work on physiological changes associated with positive emotions and positive social engagement provides some clues about how practicing positive activities improves physical health. My recent related work explores the association between positive emotions and health behavior motivation—the root of healthy lifestyles prescribed by the medical profession.

As this research evolves, collaboration between the positive psychology community and medical and health professionals will be essential. Health professionals' participation in positive psychology research is necessary to target research questions most useful to health care and toward achieving total well-being—physical, mental, psychological, and social health. Moreover, as the evidence base accumulates, positive psychologists and medical/health professionals can work together to develop and adapt best practices and tools specifically for health care settings.

Towards the aim of advancing this collaboration, the lifestyle medicine community reached out to the positive psychology and behavioral medicine communities to begin dialogue about effective early strategies to integrate the science of positive psychology into health care. I was delighted to present a keynote address at the inaugural Summit on Happiness Science in Health Care sponsored by the American College of Lifestyle Medicine and hosted by Dell Medical School in the spring of 2018. The recommendations from the Summit are being shared through publications, conference presentations, and social media discussions, propelling the movement forward.

With this work, dialogue and action towards effective integration of positive psychology interventions into healthy lifestyles and treatments are just beginning. We have much more research to conduct about the physiological changes associated with positive psychology interventions. We also need to expand translational research into health care settings to determine how health providers can leverage the lessons from basic research in practical ways.

While we are building the positive psychology evidence base for health settings, health providers can put the best and most pertinent extant research into practice. In that vein, I'm delighted that Dr. Liana Lianov, with the support of the Happiness Science and Positive Health Committee of the American College of Lifestyle Medicine, has taken the initiative to develop this handbook on positive psychology in health care. Authors in this volume discuss current research in ways that are meaningful to health providers and offer practical recommendations. This volume stands to make the reciprocal links among positive psychology, health, and health behaviors more accessible for a spectrum of health professionals. I also hope that these professionals will be inspired to use the information for their self-care, participate in research relevant to their settings, and adopt small changes in their health care practices.

I look forward to a potential new age of health care and public health that has the capacity to fully harness the discoveries from positive psychology to support total well-being for all patients, the public, and all physicians and medical/health professionals.

Barbara L. Fredrickson, Ph.D.
Kenan Distinguished Professor of Psychology and Neuroscience
University of North Carolina at Chapel Hill
Author of *Positivity* and *Love 2.0*
Past-President, International Positive Psychology Association

Preface

"A good physician treats the disease; a great physician treats the patient who has the disease."

- William Osler
Professor of Clinical Medicine
Cofounder Johns Hopkins Hospital

I'm thrilled to offer you this breakthrough book that introduces physicians and health professionals (hereinafter referred to as medical practitioners) on the relevance of positive psychology to health and health care, and how medical practices can optimally harness this key pillar of a healthy lifestyle. The information uniquely aims at reviewing the topic through the lens of the medical practitioner, but will be of interest to anyone seeking to promote their own well-being and that of others. The role of positive psychology (PP) in lifestyle medicine (LM) is highlighted, because healthy lifestyles, prescribed as the key treatment by LM practitioners, is intricately linked with positive emotion and emotional well-being. The topic addresses our shared humanity and the ultimate driver for seeking health and providing health care—to fully engage in and enjoy life, hence is relevant to all medical specialists and health professionals.

In response to requests for practical information about how to apply positive psychology in medical practice, we provide practical tips for assessing well-being, prescribing interventions, coaching health behaviors, conducting research, teaching, advocating for positive health care change, applying PP for our own well-being, and more. Busy medical practitioners can go directly to any chapter that covers their topic of choice for quick reference. For those who wish to fully implement PP, reading through all chapters is encouraged.

The recommendations are based on research conducted in a variety of settings often outside of health care, because the evidence base specific for health care settings is still being built. As research addresses unanswered questions, the implementation of PP in health care will evolve and best practices will emerge. We encourage interested practitioners to stay tuned to such developments and updates on the American College of Lifestyle Medicine website (www.lifestylemedice.org), the International Positive Psychology Association website (www.ippanetwork.org) and other credible resources listed at the end of this book. In the meantime, we hope you find this resource useful for transforming your health care practice to effectively foster total well-being through positive psychology strategies that benefit patients and practitioners alike.

With deep gratitude for your collective dedication to promoting health and happiness,
Liana Lianov, MD, MPH, FACLM, FACPM, DipABLM
Chair, Positive Health and Happiness Science Committee,
American College of Lifestyle Medicine
President, Positive Health and Wellness Division,
International Positive Psychology Association
Vice-chair, American Board of Lifestyle Medicine

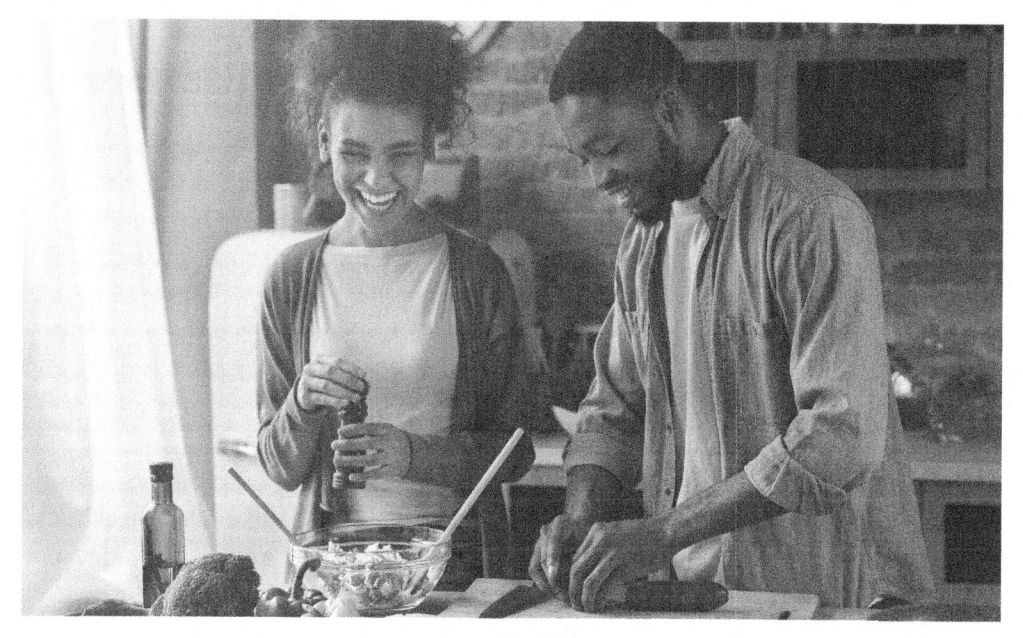

CHAPTER 1
Introduction
The Evolution of Two Interdependent Fields: Lifestyle Medicine and Positive Psychology

Chapter Goal:
To describe how positive psychology (PP) can promote effective health care practice that emphasizes healthy lifestyles for prevention and treatment, as in the field of lifestyle medicine (LM).

Chapter Highlights:
- The field of lifestyle medicine (LM) emphasizes the role of healthy lifestyles in preventing and treating disease for health and well-being.
- The field of positive psychology (PP) evolved in parallel to LM with aims to leverage individual strengths and virtues to achieve flourishing and well-being.
- The interventions of these two fields have the potential to reinforce each other for achieving well-being outcomes.
- The health professional's role in facilitating behavior change and health outcomes can be aided by leveraging PP principles and interventions.
- Not only do interventions based in PP have the potential to assist behavior change (i.e. positive emotions can boost healthy behaviors), but they can lead to direct physiological improvements.
- As the fields of LM and PP continue to evolve, closer collaboration in research and practice integration has the potential to advance both fields; future LM competencies can be revised to highlight the role of PP.

The Evolution of Lifestyle Medicine

A small group of health practitioners has been using the term "lifestyle medicine" since 1988. The American College of Lifestyle Medicine (ACLM) was founded in 2004 and defined LM as, "… the use of evidence-based lifestyle therapeutic approaches, such as predominantly whole food, plant-based diet, regular physical activity, adequate sleep, stress management, avoidance of risky substance use and other non-drug modalities, to prevent, treat, and, oftentimes, reverse lifestyle-related chronic disease" (www.lifestyle-medicine.org). However, no widely accepted definition existed until 2009, when ACLM and the American College of Preventive Medicine (ACPM) convened a panel of representatives from an array of medical specialty and health professional societies to develop a standard definition and to identify the knowledge and skill competencies physicians need in order to offer high quality lifestyle medicine services.

The definition of LM the panel developed is, "The evidence-based practice of helping individuals and families adopt and sustain healthy behaviors that affect health and quality of life" (Lianov & Johnson 2010). They also noted that this approach includes, but is not limited to, healthy eating, physical activity, sleep and avoiding risky substance use. This definition emphasizes the practitioner's role in facilitating patients' behavior change as the core of clinical practice. As health care evolves to address high costs and poor health outcomes towards a movement of value-based care, these lifestyle interventions are moving closer to center stage in a growing number of health care communities and settings beyond lifestyle medicine practice.

The lifestyle medicine national panel recommended these physician core competencies: 1) perform comprehensive lifestyle assessments, including risk factors and patient readiness to change modifiable risk factors; 2) use national guidelines in lifestyle prescriptions, when appropriate; 3) use a team approach and establish effective patient and caregiver relationships; 4) make referrals when appropriate; 5) use information technology to maximize continuity of care; 6) personally practice a healthy lifestyle and; 7) promote healthy behaviors as the foundation for clinical care and lifestyle medicine (Lianov & Johnson 2010).

The roles of health behavior change (which is closely linked to positive emotions as described in Chapter 2), emotional well-being, social support, and effective relationships are prominent elements of the competencies, and can apply not only to LM practitioners, but also other medical practitioners seeking to facilitate healthy lifestyles and improve health outcomes. Table 1 provides the complete list of the competencies, as worded by the consensus panel, and highlights the segments that relate to these elements.

Table 1: Health Behavior, Emotional Well-Being and Relationships Highlighted in the Lifestyle Medicine Core Competencies

Competency Domain	Core Competencies
Leadership	Promote **healthy behaviors as foundational** to medical care, disease prevention, and health promotion. Seek to **practice healthy behaviors** and create school, work, and home **environments that support healthy behaviors.**
Knowledge	Demonstrate knowledge of the evidence that specific **lifestyle changes** can have a positive effect on patients' health outcomes. Describe ways that **physician engagement with patients and families** can have a positive effect on patients' **health behaviors.**
Assessment Skills	Assess the **social, psychological,** and biological **predispositions of patients' behaviors** and the resulting health outcomes. Assess patient and family **readiness, willingness, and ability to make health behavior changes.** Perform a history and physical examination specific to lifestyle-related health status, including lifestyle "vital signs" such as tobacco use, alcohol consumption, diet, physical activity, body mass index, **stress level,** sleep, and **emotional well-being.** Based on this assessment, obtain and interpret appropriate tests to screen, diagnose, and monitor lifestyle-related diseases.
Management Skills	Use nationally recognized practice guidelines (such as those for hypertension and smoking cessation) to assist patients in **self-managing** their **health behaviors** and lifestyles. Establish **effective relationships** with patients and their families to effect and sustain **behavioral change** using **evidence-based counseling** methods, tools and follow-up. **Collaborate with patients and their families** to develop evidence-based, achievable, specific, written action plans such as lifestyle prescriptions. Help patients manage and **sustain healthy lifestyle practices,** and refer patients to other health care professionals as needed for lifestyle-related conditions.
Use of Office and Community Support	Have the ability to practice as an interdisciplinary team of health care professionals and support a **team approach.** Develop and apply office systems and practices to support lifestyle medical care including decision support technology. Measure processes and outcomes to improve quality of lifestyle interventions in individuals and groups of patients. Use appropriate community referral resources that support the implementation of healthy lifestyles.

This successful collaboration across a spectrum of medical and health professional societies to define LM and its core competencies was seen as a breakthrough for the field. Moreover, most of these competencies can be recognized as essential to primary care and a spectrum of specialties to achieve improved health outcomes and for health systems shifting to value-based care. Ultimately, effective health care is grounded in healthy lifestyle changes that can be facilitated by applying these competencies, the roots of which depend on behavior change driven by positive emotion and emotional well-being. Beth Frates highlights these drivers in her comprehensive and useful introduction to the LM field, *Lifestyle Medicine Handbook,* with practical recommendations in chapters on mindfulness, connection and positivity (Frates et al 2019).

The Evolution of Positive Psychology

As the field of LM was developing, a new field of psychology was being ushered into the modern era by Martin Seligman–positive psychology. This new field is defined as the scientific study of human flourishing or the strengths and virtues that enable individuals, communities and organizations to thrive; or, stated more broadly, the study of the conditions and processes that contribute to the flourishing or optimal functioning of people, groups, and institutions (Gable & Haidt 2005).

The term was coined by Abraham Maslow in 1954, who first argued that psychology was not advancing the study of human potential (Maslow 1954). Over subsequent years, other scientists showed interest; in fact, physician, philosopher and psychologist William James is considered by some as America's "first positive psychologist" due to his work on optimal human functioning. But it was Seligman, when he chose PP as the central theme for the term of his presidency of the American Psychological Association in 1998, who propelled this area of study into the limelight.

Just as LM and other medical practitioners are seeking to impact health and quality of life broadly, through healthy lifestyles, positive psychologists are seeking to promote mental health and emotional well-being beyond the absence of mental illness (Srinivasan 2015). Many outstanding researchers have contributed to the field and accelerated this work. And, in recent years many clinical counselors and psychologists have been trained in formal programs such as the University of Pennsylvania's Masters in Applied Positive Psychology (MAPP) program.

The fields of LM and PP progressed in parallel without much cross-discipline collaboration. Yet the interventions offered by each field have the potential to reinforce each other to achieve desired health outcomes. The need for accelerating the integration of the principles and science of the fields became clearly apparent during a 2017 keynote address by one of the leading PP researchers, Barbara Fredrickson, then president of the International Positive Psychology Association (IPPA), at IPPA's 5th World Congress in Montreal. Her presentation emphasized the role of positive affect in lifestyle behaviors. Health behaviors can be influenced by positive psychological approaches, not only when PP is applied with behavior change coaching/counseling techniques, such as motivational interviewing, but also when positive affect, especially when associated with that behavior, drives unconscious motivation for change (Van Cappellen et al 2018). This research has not been widely shared with the health care community, even in the face of continuing challenges to support patients in achieving and sustaining healthy lifestyle changes.

To promote well-being and health, medical practitioners need to address mental, emotional and social health, as well as physical health. Leveraging research-informed PP principles has the potential to improve each of these health elements, and to promote an additional, independent element of health–positive health. The term positive health was coined by Seligman to signify a health attribute (with biological, subjective and functional elements) that produces longer, healthier life, and lowers disease risk factors over and above what is accomplished by traditional health care (Seligman 2008).

In response to this need to expand awareness, education and training about PP to medical practitioners, ACLM convened the Happiness Science and Positive Health Committee. The Committee aims to advance the integration of science-based PP into health care practice through reviewing and aggregating the science most relevant to health and health care, developing training programs and tools, and engaging champions across a variety of health care settings who can collaborate on research to produce a clear evidence base and best practices. This handbook is an early tool that will be updated as the research and the field evolve.

Terms and Definitions

Psychologists and medical practitioners have not yet reached consensus on definitions for a range of terms used to refer to states of happiness and well-being. Examples include subjective well-being, psychological well-being, happiness, resiliency, and flourishing. In this book, we use the term **healthy lifestyle** to refer to physical habits that can lead to health and well-being. We use **positive psychology interventions (PPIs)** for intentional (whether self-selected or prescribed by a professional) strategies, activities and behaviors that can lead to positive affect and psychological states and, in turn, are associated with healthy behavior changes and physiologic benefits. We use the term **total well-being** to include, not only those health areas in the World Health Organization's definition of health (https://www.who.int), but also Seligman's areas of positive health:

- Physical health–absence of physical risk factors and disease
- Mental health–absence of mental illness
- Emotional health–ability to cope with stress, normal self-confidence and self-esteem, resilience, optimism, ability to learn and adapt and to be flexible
- Social health–having healthy relationships
- Positive health–health asset leading to greater health and longer life achieved by behaviors based in the science of positive psychology

We also use the term **emotional well-being** for combined states of emotional and positive health.

Some individuals might be concerned that the PP focus could lead to "Pollyanna-ish" thinking and suppression of negative emotions. However, when promoting total well-being with a positive psychology approach, individuals need to be encouraged to embrace negative feelings as well as positive ones. In fact, experiencing a broad spectrum of emotions, called emodiversity, is healthy (Ong et al 2018).

The Reinforcing Nature of Healthy Lifestyles and Positive Psychology

The implementation of PP strategies by medical practitioners to assist health behavior coaching and the inclusion of PPIs in treatment plans can potentially have significant benefits. Chapter 2 reviews the salient studies that demonstrate the reinforcing relationship between PP and healthy lifestyles. Benefits of PPIs include emotional well-being and increased capacity to build supportive resources (Cohn & Fredrickson 2010; Fredrickson 2013; Fredrickson et al 2008; Kok & Fredrickson 2010; Kok et al 2013; Redwine et al 2016), adherence to healthy behaviors (Gardner et al 2014, Van Cappellen et al 2018), greater health outcomes (Cohen et al 2016; Kubzansky et al 2018; Yeung et al 2018), decreased health care utilization (Kim et al 2013), increased preventive care (Kim et al 2014), and increased longevity (Chida & Steptoe 2008; Danner et al 2001; Eichstaedt et al 2015). Wound healing, inflammation, immunity (Pressman & Black 2012; Brod et al 2014), telomere length (Blackburn 2018; Puterman & Epel 2012), and endocrine and gene regulation (Nelson-Coffey et al 2017) are among some of the physical processes and pathways that may account for the impact of positive emotion on health. Even fleeting positive "micro-moments" of connectivity contribute to well-being and health (Sandstrom & Dunn 2014).

The reverse is also true. Evidence suggests engaging in healthy behaviors contributes to enhanced positive emotions and states. For example, individuals who exercise and eat a diet high in vegetables report greater happiness (Jacka 2010, 2011); moreoever self-reported happiness influences food choice (Gardner et al 2014). In fact, every major healthy lifestyle modality, (e.g., eating a whole food plant-based diet, being physically active, getting adequate and high quality sleep, and avoiding risky substance use), has this reciprocal relationship with positive emotion, as described in Chapter 2. Hence, the dynamic and multiplicative impact of healthy lifestyle and habits based in PP that promotes total well-being deserves much more attention in health care settings.

Many questions remain to be answered in order to build the evidence base on how best to apply the principles of PP and use PPIs in health care settings. We briefly summarize the state of current research, as well as research gaps, in Chapter 11. Moreover, the study of PP, as with other psychology subfields, has complexities and nuances that need to be sorted out in order to develop customized interventions that are more likely to be effective in particular patient populations. We review some of these nuances in Chapter 7. One essential consideration is the aim of a specific treatment plan or intervention. Different recommendations and standards will likely evolve for different aims, among them emotional well-being, quality of life, coping with pain and recovery from illness, physical health and longevity. Leaders and medical practitioners in the movement to closely integrate PP and health care need to work with behavioral researchers to identify and appropriately frame these and other research questions.

Future Vision: Highlighting Positive Psychology in Lifestyle Medicine and Beyond

Given the significant role PPIs may play in achieving a spectrum of health care aims, LM core competencies can be adjusted to emphasize this role in support of promoting high quality care. Table 2 highlights the existing competencies that relate to or are impacted by PP and offers recommendations for PP specific additions (in bold). Future revisions or expansions of the competencies might include such additions. In the meantime, medical practitioners interested in enhancing their practices with PP strategies may consider using these recommendations as a guide.

Table 2: Lifestyle Medicine Core Competencies: Highlighting and Expanding the Role of Positive Psychology

Competency Domain	Core Competencies
Leadership	Promote **physical and psychological health behaviors** as foundational to medical care, disease prevention, health promotion, and total **well-being (physical, mental, psychological, social, and positive health)**. Seek to **practice physical and psychological health behaviors** and create school, work, and home environments that support healthy behaviors.
Knowledge	Demonstrate knowledge of the evidence that specific **lifestyle changes, facilitated by social support and positive emotion,** can have a positive effect on patients' health outcomes. Describe ways that **physician engagement with patients and families,** including **demonstration of empathy and conducting positive interactions,** can have a positive effect on patients' health behaviors.
Assessment Skills	**Assess the social, psychological,** and biological **predispositions of patients' behaviors** and the resulting health outcomes. Assess patient and family **readiness, willingness, and ability to make health behavior changes, and assess social, psychological and emotional resources and supports for making changes.** Perform a history and physical examination specific to lifestyle-related health status, including lifestyle "vital signs" such as tobacco use, alcohol consumption, diet, physical activity, body mass index, stress level, sleep, **and positive activities (based on the science of positive psychology).** Based on this assessment, obtain and interpret appropriate tests to screen, diagnose, and monitor lifestyle-related diseases.
Management Skills	Use nationally recognized practice guidelines (such as those for hypertension and smoking cessation) to assist patients in **self-managing** their **health behaviors** and lifestyles. Establish **effective relationships** with patients and their families to effect and sustain **behavioral change** using **evidence-based counseling methods, including motivational interviewing, cognitive behavioral and positive psychology techniques,** tools and follow-up. **Collaborate with patients and their families** to develop evidence-based, achievable, specific, written action plans, such as lifestyle prescriptions that address major elements of a healthy lifestyle, **including physical, social, and psychological behaviors/activities.** Help patients manage and **sustain healthy lifestyle practices,** and refer patients to other health care professionals as needed for lifestyle-related conditions.

Use of Office and Community Support	Have the ability to practice as an interdisciplinary team of health care professionals and support a **team approach.**
	Develop and apply office systems and practices to support lifestyle medical care including decision support technology.
	Measure processes and outcomes to improve quality of lifestyle interventions in individuals and groups of patients.
	Use appropriate community referral resources that support the implementation of healthy lifestyles, **including digital technology/mobile apps that support total well-being.**

These recommended revisions to the original competencies are not formally adopted at the time of this writing. With the recent inclusion of PP in the American Board of Lifestyle Medicine (ABLM) certification examination and in LM trainings, the topic of PP is gaining greater recognition as an essential competency area. Emphasis will likely grow as the broader health care community recognizes the integral role of PP in promoting healthy lifestyle behaviors, its physiologic benefits, its role in total well-being, and the emerging research on positive health (that results from positive emotions and activities) as an additional pillar of health.

Summary

The fields of LM and PP have evolved independently, yet science suggests they have the potential to reinforce and accelerate their common goal of promoting total well-being. By embracing PP principles and strategies, the health care community can achieve multiple goals, including:

- Promote total well-being of patients with all key elements of a healthy lifestyle, including emotional well-being
- Engage in positive and effective patient-provider interactions
- Manage mental illness and promote mental health; e.g., ameliorate depression associated with chronic disease, and enhance or supplement treatment of mental illness
- Coach for health behaviors more effectively by enhancing coaching approaches, such as motivational interviewing, with PP approaches
- Drive unconscious motivation for healthy habits
- Promote beneficial physiologic effects
- Improve quality of life
- Develop effective and satisfying medical practices

Table 3 summarizes the potential role of PP in health care by highlighting overarching goals that can be addressed with PP strategies, key processes and mechanisms that PP offers to help achieve those goals, and future tasks the health care community needs to accomplish (in collaboration with the PP community) in order to optimize health care with PP.

Table 3: The Role of Positive Psychology (PP) in Health Care

Health Care Goals	Processes/Mechanisms	Future Tasks
Promote total well-being of patients	Boost positive emotion	Develop consistent terminology and measurement
Enhance health behavior coaching	Support positive, empathetic and effective patient-provider interactions	Disseminate PP science, training and tools
Increase motivation for healthy habits	Integrate PP with motivational interviewing and cognitive behavioral techniques	Conduct PP translational research in health care settings
Improve quality of life	Drive unconscious motivation	Develop best practice guidelines for use of PP in health care
Increase satisfaction and well-being of medical practitioners	Promote beneficial physiologic effects	Enhance capacity of health systems (payment, digital technology, human resources) to address total well-being, including positive health
	Address mental illness; e.g., ameliorate depression associated with chronic diseases	

References

American College of Lifestyle Medicine, www.lifestylemedicine.org

Blackburn E. *The Telomere Effect: A Revolutionary Approach to Living Younger, Healthier, Longer.* New York City, New York: Grand Central Publishing, 2018.

Brod S, Rattazzi L, Piras G, et al. 'As above, so below' examining the interplay between emotion and the immune system. *Immunology* 2014;143:311-318. doi:10.1111/imm.12341.

Chida Y, Steptoe A. Positive psychological well-being and mortality: a qualitative review of perspective observational studies. *Psychosom Med.* 2008;70:741-756.

Cohn MA, Fredrickson BL. In search of durable positive psychology interventions: Predictors and consequences of long-term positive behaviour change. *J Posit Psychol.* 2010;5(5):355-366.

Cohen R, Bavishi C, Rozanski A. Purpose in life and its relationship to all-cause mortality and cardiovascular events: a meta-analysis. *Psychosom Med.* 2016;78(2):122-133

Danner DD, Snowden DA, Friesen WV. Positive emotions in early life and longevity: findings from the nun study. *J Pers Soc Psychol.* 2001; 80(5):804-813.

Eichstaedt JC, Schwartz HA, Kern ML, et al. Psychological language on twitter predicts county-level heart disease mortality. *Psychol Sci.* 2015;26(2):159-169. doi:10.1177/0956797614557867.

Frates B, Bonnet JP, Joseph R, Peterson JA. *Lifestyle Medicine Handbook, An Introduction to the Power of Healthy Habits.* Monterey, CA: Healthy Living, 2019.

Fredrickson BL. Positive emotions broaden and build. *Adv Exp Soc Psychol.* 2013;47:1-53.

Fredrickson BL, Cohn MA, Coffey KA, et al. Open hearts build lives: Positive emotions, induced through loving-kindness meditation, build consequential personal resources. *J Pers Soc Psychol.* 2008;92:1045-1062.

Gable SL, Haidt J. What (and Why) is positive psychology? *Rev Gen Psychol.* 9(2):103-110.

Gardner MP, Wansink B, Kim J, et al. Better moods for better eating? How mood influences food choice. *J Consumer Psychol.* 2014;24(3):320-335.

Jacka FN. Association of Western and traditional diets with depression and anxiety in women. *Am J Psychiat.* 2010;167:305-511.

Jacka FN. The association between habitual diet quality and the common mental disorders in communit-dwelling adults: the Hordaland Health Study. *Psychosom. Med.* 2011;73(6):483-490.

Kim ES, Sun JK, Park N, et al. Purpose in life and reduced risk of myocardial infarction among older US adults with coronary heart disease: a two-year follow-up. *J Behav Med.* 2013;36(2):124-133.

Kim ES, Strecher VJ, Ryff CD. Purpose in life and use of preventive health care services. *Proc Natl Acad Sci.* 2014;111(46):16331-16336.

Kok BE, Coffey KA, Cohn MA, et al. How positive emotions build physical health: perceived positive social connections account for the upward spiral between positive emotions and vagal tone. *Psychol Sci.* 2013;24:1123-1132.

Kok BE, Fredrickson BL. Upward spirals of the heart: Autonomic flexibility, as indexed by vagal tone, reciprocally and prospectively predicts positive emotions and social connectedness. *Biol Psychol.* 2010;85:432-436.

Kubzansky LD, Huffman JC, Boehm JK, et al. Positive psychological well-being and cardiovascular disease. JACC health promotion series. *J Am Coll Cardiol.* 2018;72(12), 1382-1396.

Lianov L, Johnson M. Physician competencies for prescribing lifestyle medicine. *JAMA.* 2010;304(2):202-203.

Maslow AH. *Motivation and Personality.* New York: Harper, 1954, p.354.

Nelson-Coffey K, Fritz MM, Lyubomirsky S, et al. Kindness in the blood: A randomized controlled trial of the gene regulatory impact of prosocial behavior. *Psychoneuroendocrinol.* 2017;81:8-13.

Ong AD, Benson L, Zautra, AJ, et al. Emodiversity and biomarkers of inflammation. *Emotion* 2018;18(1):3-14. doi:10.1037/emo0000343 https://www.emodiversity.org/findings; accessed April 12, 2019.

Pressman SD, Black LL. Positive Emotions and Immunity. In Segerstrom SC. Oxford University Press USA: *The Oxford Handbook of Psychoneuroimmunology,* 2012.

Puterman E. Epel E. An intricate dance: Life experience, multisystem resiliency, and rate of telomere decline throughout the lifespan. *Soc Pers Psychol Compass.* 2012;6(11).

Redwine LS, Henry BS, Pung MA, et al. J Pilot Randomized Study of a Gratitude Journaling Intervention on heart rate variability and inflammatory biomarkers in patients with stage B heart failure. *Psychosom Med.* 2016 Jul-Aug;78(6):667-76.

Sandstrom GM, Dunn EW. Social interactions and well-being. The surprising power of weak ties. *Pers Soc Psychol B.* 2014;40, 910-922.

Selgman MEP. Positive Health. *Appl Psychol.* 2008;57(s1).

Srinivasan TS. The 5 Founding Fathers and History of Positive Psychology, Positive Psychology Program, Feb 12, 2015.

Van Cappellen P, Rice EL, Catalino LI, et al. Positive affective processes underlie positive health behavior change. *Psychol Health* 2018;33:77-97.

World Health Organizaiton: https://www.who.int/

Yeung JWK, Zhang Z, Kim TY. Volunteering and health benefits in general adults: cumulative effects and forms. *BMC Public Health* 2018;18:8.

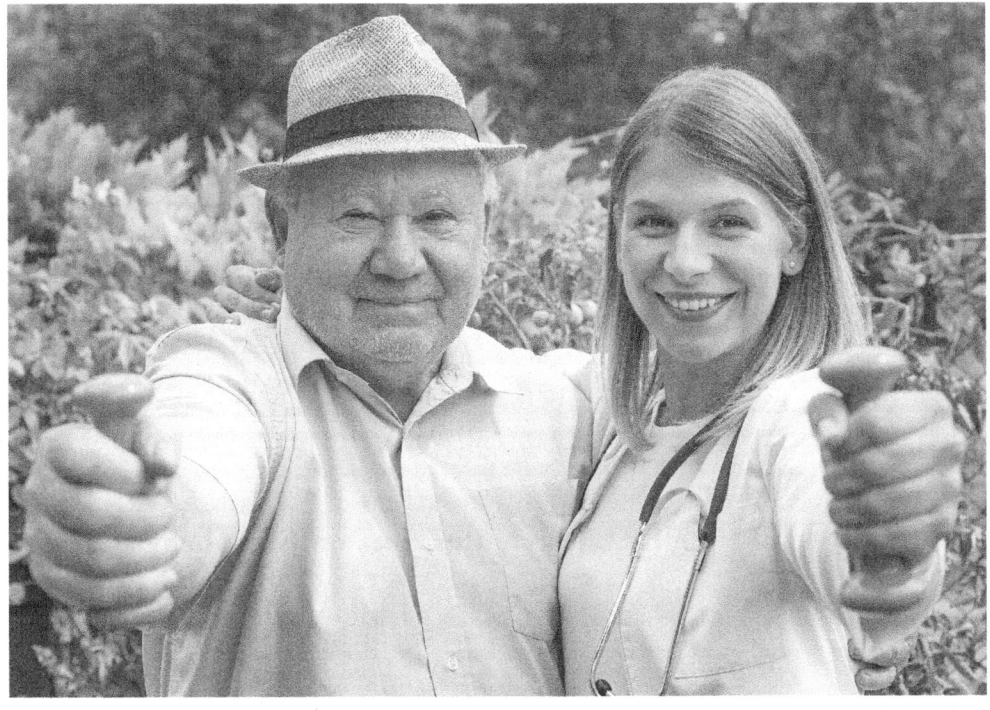

CHAPTER 2
Healthy Lifestyle Practices and Emotional Well-Being:
A Reciprocal Relationship
Darren Morton

Chapter Goal:
To describe key studies that demonstrate the reciprocal relationship between healthy lifestyle practices, positive psychology strategies and emotional well-being.

Chapter Highlights:
- Research suggests that healthy lifestyles, namely a predominantly plant-based diet, exercise, and sleep, are associated with self-reports of feeling better emotionally.
- Time in nature is also associated with improved mood and physiology, such as greater heart rate variability (HRV), which can lead to better health outcomes.
- Positive psychology activities, such as practicing gratitude, have been associated with: fewer strokes and myocardial infarctions; lower body mass index, lipids, HgbA1C and insulin resistance; and better HRV.
- Social connectivity, leading to positive emotions and "positive resonance," is an additional and essential element of emotional well-being.
- Studies suggest that positive affect is associated with positive health behaviors. Hence, healthy behaviors and activities that boost positive affect can have a reciprocal relationship.

A Reciprocal Relationship

Healthy lifestyle choices are established protective factors for a myriad of physical ailments, such as heart disease and type 2 diabetes, and can even be viable treatment options (Ford et al 2009, Lean et al 2018, Ornish et al 1990). While the causal link between a healthy lifestyle and physical health is well-established, there is a growing body of evidence that healthy lifestyle practices also confer mental health and emotional well-being benefits. Studies suggest that positive lifestyle choices such as healthy eating, exercise, sleep and exposure to nature effectively reduce negative affect and promote positive affect. In other words, practicing healthy behaviors may alleviate depression and help happiness. Notably, just as healthy behaviors can help individuals experience more positive emotions, there is evidence that suggests positive emotions may drive healthier behaviors (Van Cappellen et al 2018), resulting in better health outcomes. Indeed, the relationship between healthy lifestyle practices and emotional well-being is reciprocal.

The Influence of Healthy Lifestyle Practices on Emotional Well-Being

Virtually every major healthy lifestyle practice has beneficial effects on emotional well-being.

Healthy Nutrition

The influence of food on mood is attracting extensive research attention and there is now a well-established association between diet quality and mental health (Jacka 2010, 2011; Lai et al 2014; Sanchez-Villegas et al 2010; Sanchez-Villegas 2012). Further, there is considerable evidence that nutrition interventions can reduce depressive symptoms (Aggarwal et al 2015; Beezhold & Johnston 2012; Jacka et al 2017; Parletta et al 2017) and that this may be mediated through the gut microbiota (Valles-Colmer et al 2019).

In a study by Jacka and colleagues (2017), moderately to severely depressed individuals were randomly assigned to two groups: dietary intervention (a Mediterranean-style eating pattern) with social support or social support only. Remission of depression was observed in 32% of the participants in the dietary intervention group as compared to only 8% of the participants in the social support only group. In another study of similar design, Parletta and team (2017) observed that reductions in depression were significantly correlated to participants' adherence to a Mediterranean-style eating pattern, as well as their consumption of nuts and vegetable diversity. Both these studies point to the potential benefits of diets high in plants for the management and treatment of depression. Similarly, Beezhold (2010) randomized omnivores to a control group (no change in diet), pesco-vegetarian diet or total vegetarian diet for two weeks and reported that improvements in mood only occurred among the total vegetarian group.

While the benefits of a healthy diet for alleviating negative affect are increasingly recognized, there is also growing evidence that a diet comprising of whole, plant-based foods may increase positive affect (Beezhold et al 2010; Beezhold et al 2015; Blanchflower et al 2013; Gardner et al 2013). A large epidemiological study of over 80,000 individuals in the United Kingdom observed a dose-response relationship between the consumption of fruits and vegetables and happiness, even after controlling for numerous confounding factors known to influence emotional well-being (Blanchflower et al 2013). Optimal levels of emotional well-being were reported among individuals consuming approximately 7 to 8 servings of fruits and vegetables each day. These findings concur with those of a smaller longitudinal study in which the highest levels of subjective well-being were reported by individuals consuming 8 or more servings of fruits and vegetables daily (White et al 2013). However, the science on the link between healthy food consumption and levels of emotional and subjective well-being is relatively new; hence more research is needed to determine the nature and extent of the relationship.

Physical Activity

Several reviews and Cochrane reports conclude that regular physical activity is strongly associated with better mood and prevention of depression (Cooney et al 2013; Eriksson & Gard 2011; Mammen & Faulkner 2013; Rimer et al 2012). This relationship is found among both the young (McKercher et al 2013) and the elderly (Mara & Carta 2013). Indeed, studies have even shown that exercise is comparable to antidepressant medication for relieving depression (Blumenthal et al 2007) and that exercise intervention performs significantly better than medication for preventing depression relapse (Babyak et al 2000).

Physiological, biochemical and psychological mechanisms have been proposed to explain the mood-enhancing properties of physical activity, including increases in beta-endorphins and other neurotransmitters, increased thermogenesis, regulation of the hypothalamic-pituitary-adrenal axis, increased neurogenesis, psychological distraction and improved self-efficacy (Boecker et al 2008; Ernst et al 2006; Mikkelsen et al 2017). Regardless of the mechanism, physical activity is one of the most evidence-based, effective methods available for preventing affective disorders and enhancing emotional well-being, and therefore may constitute one of the most effective and yet least utilized antidepressants available.

Few studies have examined the dose of exercise required to evoke positive affect benefits. Ekkekakis (2000) found that 10-15 minutes of walking was sufficient to improve positive affect. Hansen and colleagues (2001) examined shifts in mood following 10, 20 and 30 minutes of moderate-intensity physical activity and found that 10 minutes of exercise conferred the same improvements in mood as the longer durations. A limitation of these studies is that they did not test the effect on mood of exercise durations less than 10 minutes, and hence it is possible that even less than 10 minutes is required to induce positive emotional states.

Regarding exercise intensity, most studies to date have examined the impact of moderate aerobic exercise on mental health, but there is emerging evidence that higher intensity aerobic exercise and resistance exercise may confer additional mood-enhancing benefits (Singh et al 2005; Stanton et al 2013). However, more research is required to better understand the influence of different forms of exercise on mental health as well as optimal dosages and durations.

While the benefits of exercise for affective disorders is well documented, fewer studies have examined the ability of exercise to promote positive affect. In a cross-sectional study involving 15 European countries, higher physical activity levels were associated with greater levels of happiness, suggesting a dose-response relationship (Richards et al 2015). A confounding factor is that happier people might be more inclined to exercise. Cambridge researchers used a smartphone app to collect physical activity and happiness data on over 10,000 individuals (Lathia et al 2017). The participants reported feeling happier in the moments they were more active. The findings suggested that not only exercise, but also non-exercise physical activity may elevate moods related to happiness.

Sleep

A variety of studies have demonstrated that insomnia is a predictor of depression in subsequent years (Riemann & Voderholzer 2003). Neckelmann (2007) not only showed that lack of sleep is associated with depression and anxiety states, but also that insomnia is a risk factor for anxiety disorders. Given the deleterious impact of sleep restriction on mental health, it is alarming that at least one third of adults fail to meet the National Sleep Foundation's guidelines of 7 to 9 hours of sleep per night (Hirshkowitz et al 2015). Contributors to the high prevalence of sleep disorders may include the widespread downturn in physical activity levels, increasing use of caffeine, and increased exposure to "night light pollution" (Bedrosian & Nelson 2013). Over 99% of the world's population is exposed to artificial light at night, which may result in circadian entrainment and compromised sleep duration and quality (Bedrosian & Nelson 2013). Intriguingly, satellite imaging indicates that global luminescence increases by approximately 2% each year (Kyba et al 2017). The sleep hygiene of young adults, especially adolescents, may be particularly suffering due to widespread smart phone usage (Demirci et al 2015; Gradisar et al 2013).

Several studies have shown that even acute sleep deprivation results in the human brain being more attuned to negativity. For example, Yoo and associates observed through *f*MRI that individuals demonstrate higher levels of emotional reactivity when sleep-deprived (Yoo et al 2007). Similarly, Strickgold (2015) reported that during a memory task, sleep-deprived individuals were more than twice as likely to remember words with negative connotations compared to when they were well rested. In conclusion, quality sleep is a cornerstone of emotional well-being.

Exposure to Nature

One hundred years ago Sir John Thompson warned that increasing modernization would disconnect us from natural environments and that we would suffer for it. It would seem his words were prophetic, as there is a growing literature showing a connection between exposure to nature and mental health. This connection is not surprising given that humans have inhabited natural environments for millennia; the built environment is the newcomer.

A meta-analysis of 32 studies concluded that exposure to natural environments leads to less negative affect and greater positive affect (McMahon & Estes 2015). It seems that there is merit to "nature therapy," such as the Japanese practice *shinrin-yoko* [forest bathing]. A New Zealand study showed that every 1% increase in the amount of green space within a 2-mile radius of an individual's home was associated with a 4% lower prevalence of anxiety and mood disorders (Nutsford et al 2013). Further, exposure to "green" areas has been associated with less aggression, and even a window view of nature is significantly correlated to lower levels of domestic violence (Kuo & Sullivan 2001). For many years it has been recognized that hospital patients who have a view of a natural landscape tend to consume less painkilling medication and have shorter hospital stays (Urlich 1984). These studies testify to the impact of natural environments on mental health and well-being.

There are several theories for why nature might confer health benefits and have a calming effect (Kuo 2015). One theory suggests that modern living makes high demands of our information-processing skills, which leads to unnatural mental strain (Kaplan 1995). Conversely, natural stimuli, such as landscapes and animals, effortlessly engage our attention, leading to less mental fatigue (Pearson & Craig 2014).

One aspect of natural environments that seems to be especially important for the promotion of mental health is the intensity of the light to which individuals are exposed. Seasonal affective disorder (SAD) is a well-documented condition experienced by individuals enduring extended periods of low lighting during the winter months in countries of high latitude (Vyssoki et al 2012). SAD is characterized by low mood, depression and even suicidal inclination. Interestingly, bright light therapy is being used as a treatment for depression (Tuunainen et al 2010) and it has been found to be as effective for relieving depression as antidepressant medications (Lam et al 2016). Bright light therapy involves exposure to 10,000 lux–an intensity of light typically only found outside in naturally lit environments–for at least 30 minutes. Researchers from the University of Colorado monitored how much light individuals were exposed to on a typical day of modern living (i.e. predominately exposed to artificial light) and compared it to exposure while camping in winter (i.e. predominately exposed to natural light). During waking hours, the participants were, on average, exposed to light levels 13 times higher when camping (approximately 10,000 lux) as compared to modern living (approximately 750 lux) (Stothard et al 2016).

As individuals increasingly engage in screen-based activities and the evidence continues to accumulate showing a link between health and connection to nature, exposure to nature should be considered a more frontline therapy for affective disorders and the promotion of emotional well-being.

The Influence of Emotional Well-Being on Health Behaviors and Health Outcomes

Most people know from personal experience that their emotional state influences their lifestyle choices. Often, the reason why we don't do what we know we should–like exercise and eat healthily–is because we don't *feel* like it. Similarly, the reason we tend to do the things we know we shouldn't–like eat junk food and use substances–is because we do *feel* like it. Indeed, our emotional state can have a pronounced influence on our health behaviors and subsequent health outcomes, which presents an ongoing challenge for health care providers.

Emotional Well-Being and Health Behaviors

Gardner and colleagues (2019) showed in a series of studies that negative emotional states tend to drive behaviors that offer immediate rewards. For example, high levels of negative affect increased appetite for indulgent foods. While there is considerable evidence that poor mental health and negative emotional states can drive poor lifestyle choices (Tanihata et al 2015; Velten et al 2014), of greater interest here is the potential that positive affect may drive positive lifestyle choices (Tugade et al 2004, Van Cappellen et al 2018). This is a pertinent topic, as there is extensive evidence that positive emotion can be fostered through a variety of positive psychology interventions such as practicing mindfulness, savoring, expressing gratitude, reflecting on good experiences, supporting others, developing a sense of agency, and nurturing a sense of meaning and life purpose (Emmons & McCullough 2003, Hendriks et al 2019).

Studies show that positive psychology interventions prompt engagement in healthy eating and physical activity (Van Cappellen et al 2018) and lead to increased utilization of preventive services (Kim et al 2014). Moreover, people who report having a greater frequency of "happy moments" are more likely to exercise, not smoke, use seat belts, eat well, drink alcohol in moderation, stay married, demonstrate prosocial behaviors and work more productively (Diener & Chan 2011). Indeed, positive emotion can forecast behavioral engagement in healthy lifestyle practices, even 15 months later (Cohn & Fredrickson 2010; Rhodes & Kates 2015).

What are the mechanisms by which positive affect nudges healthy behavior change? According to the seminal work of leading researcher, Barbara Fredrickson, positive emotion builds nonconscious motivation—a natural, inner, non-imposed desire for change (Fredrickson 2013). This "upward spiral theory" describes a reinforcing phenomenon through which pleasant, intrinsic and natural emotions increase motivation and positive health behaviors by activating thought-action repertoires that lead to exploring and trying new things, which, in turn, builds an individual's physical, psychological and social resources (Catalino & Fredrickson 2011; Fredrickson et al 2008; Van Cappellen et al 2018). In brief, positive emotion broadens awareness, receptivity, creativity and problem solving capacity. Combined with greater self-efficacy, self-control and cognitive capacity, these resources may improve the likelihood of coping successfully when challenges arise (Fredrickson 2004; 2015; Kok & Fredrickson 2010; Kok et al 2013).

Given the contribution of positive emotion to healthy lifestyle behaviors, it is encouraging that positive psychology approaches are increasingly being weaved into behavior change counseling, such as motivational interviewing and cognitive behavioral techniques. There is a need for more health care providers to be aware of and intentionally use positive psychology strategies to leverage positive affect as a direct tool to spur motivation and behavior change.

Emotional Well-Being and Health Outcomes

As discussed above, positive affect may have the potential to drive positive health behaviors and hence it is unremarkable that numerous studies have shown an association between positive psychology approaches and better health outcomes. Sustained gratitude and mindfulness practices, as well as activities that promote a sense of meaning and life purpose, have been associated with fewer strokes and myocardial infarctions; lower body mass index, lipids, HgbA1C and insulin resistance; and better heart rate variability (Huffman et al 2015; Kim et al 2013; Kim et al 2014; Redwine et al 2016).

The association of positive mindset and emotional states with health outcomes can be powerful. For example, Eichstaedt and colleagues analyzed the word choices used in approximately 150 million Twitter posts originating from numerous locations around the United States and found positive word choice to be significantly correlated with lower regional prevalence of cardiovascular mortality (Eichstaedt et al 2015). Indeed, several studies have reported emotional well-being to be a significant contributor to longevity—even more influential than many other well-established predictors including income, education, physical activity level and smoking status (Chida & Steptoe 2008). A landmark study that followed nuns over their lives showed that those who were rated the happiest, according to the level of optimism and positivity in their early life writings, lived about six years longer (Danner et al 2001). Other studies have confirmed this association between survival and positive affect (Chida & Steptoe 2008).

Moreover, positive emotions arising from social connectivity have been shown to correlate with physiologic benefits, such as improved cardiac vagal tone and increased heart rate variability (Kok & Fredrickson 2010). Surprisingly, even weak social ties and micromoments of connection with strangers can positively influence a variety of health metrics including telomere length and lifespan (Isgett et al 2017; Major et al 2018; Mathur et al 2016; Nelson-Coffey et al 2017; Sandstrom & Dunn 2014; Waugh & Fredrickson 2006). Helping patients understand these effects might spur them to create more positive brief social connections, such as offering authentic, kind greetings to people they encounter throughout the day. Acts of kindness are also linked to positive health benefits. In one study, participants who were randomized to engage in acts of kindness toward others experienced a shift in gene expression associated with anti-inflammation (Nelson-Coffey et al 2017).

In conclusion, promoting positive affect and emotional well-being can provide many benefits. Importantly, these benefits are available to both patients and providers. In the interest of self-care, health care providers can harness lifestyle and positive psychology strategies to enhance and sustain their personal well-being.

Summary

This chapter has highlighted some of the ways that a healthy lifestyle improves emotional well-being and boosts positive emotions and vitality. Selected studies are listed in Table 1. It has also explored how positive emotional states can reciprocally drive and support healthy lifestyle behaviors (and associated outcomes). These observations point to the importance of promoting psychological health and emotional well-being, and including positive psychology-based activities as a cornerstone of overall health care.

Table 1: Summary of Selected Studies

Author (Year)	Study design/setting	Participants	Conclusion
Agarwal et al (2015)	Quasi-experimental (intervention and control groups)	292 participants in a workplace setting	A plant-based diet program resulted in significantly greater improvements in depression and workplace productivity.
Beezhold & Johnston (2012)	RCT.	39 omnivores	Restricting meat, fish and poultry improved domains of mood.
Blanchflower et al. (2013)	Cross-sectional study	80,000 British adults	Happiness and mental health rise in approximately dose-response relationship with fruit and vegetable consumption. 7-8 serves optimal.
Blumenthal et al (2007)	Prospective RCT	202 patients with diagnosis of depression	An exercise intervention was as comparable for relieving depression as antidepressant medication.
Jacka et al (2017)	RCT	67 patients with diagnosis of depression	A 12-week Mediterranean-style dietary intervention was four times more effective for depression remission.
Lam et al (2016)	Randomized, double-blinded, placebo and sham controlled	122 patients with non-seasonal major depressive disorder	Eight weeks of "bright light therapy" was more effective than fluoxetine for depression remission.
Parletta et al (2017)	RCT	152 individuals with self-diagnosed depression	Adherence to a Mediterranean-style diet supplemented with fish oil resulted in significant reductions in depression and improved mental health over 6 months.
Richards et al (2015)	Epidemiological	11,637 individuals from 15 European countries	Increasing physical activity volume was associated with higher levels of happiness.
Sandstrom & Dunn (2013)	Randomized comparative study	60 community-based individuals	Social interaction with a "weak social tie" (e.g. barista) promoted positive affect, which was mediated by feelings of belonging.
Singh et al (2005)	RCT	60 older (>60 yrs.) community-dwelling individuals with major or minor depression	High-intensity resistance exercise was more effective than low-intensity exercise for treating depression.
Van Cappellen et al (2018)	Series of four studies		Study outcomes supported an "upward spiral theory of lifestyle change" in which positive emotion promotes healthy lifestyle choices.

References

Aggarwal U, Mishra S, Xu J, et al. A multicenter randomized controlled trial of a nutrition intervention program in a multiethnic adult population in the corporate settings reduces depression and anxiety and improved quality of life: the GEICO study. *Am J Health Promot*. 2015; 29(4):245-54.

Babyak M, Blumenthal JA, Herman S, et al. Exercise Treatment for Major Depression: Maintenance of Therapeutic Benefit at 10 Months. *Psychosom Med.* 2000;62:633–638.

Bedrosian TA, Nelson RJ. Influence of the modern light environment on mood. *Molecul Psychiat.* 2013;18(7):751-757.

Beezhold BL, Johnston CS, Daigle DR. Vegetarian diets are associated with healthy mood states: a cross-sectional study in Seventh Day Adventist adults. *Nut. J.* 2010;1:9-26.

Beezhold BL, Johnston CS. Restriction of meat, fish, ad poultry in omnivores improves mood: a pilot randomized controlled trial. *Nutr J.* 2012;11:9.

Beezhold B, Radnitz C, Rinne A, DiMatteo J. Vegans report less stress and anxiety. *Nutr Neurosci.* 2015;18(7):289-96.

Blanchflower D, Oswald A, Stewart-Brown S. Is psychological wellbeing linked to the consumption of fruit and vegetables? *Soc Indic Res.* 2013;114:785-801.

Blumenthal JA, Babyak MA, Doraiswamy PM, et al. Exercise and pharmacotherapy in the treatment of major depressive disorder. *Psychosom Med.* 2007;69(7):587-596.

Boecker H, Sprenger T, Spilker ME, et al. The runner's high: opioidergic mechanisms in the human brain. *Cereb Cortex.* 2008;18(11):2523-2531.

Catalino LI, Fredrickson BL. A Tuesday in the life of a flourisher: The role of positive emotional reactivity in optimal mental health. *Emotion.* 2011;11:938-950.

Chida Y, Steptoe A. Positive psychological well-being and mortality: a qualitative review of perspective observational studies. *Psychosom Med.* 2008;70:741-756.

Cohn MA, Fredrickson BL. In search of durable positive psychology interventions: Predictors and consequences of long-term positive behaviour change. *J Posit Psychol.* 2010;5(5):355-366.

Cooney GM, Dwan K, Greig CA, et al. Exercise for depression, *Cochrane Database Syst Rev.* 2013;9.

Danner DD, Snowden DA, Friesen WV. Positive emotions in early life and longevity: findings from the nun study. *J Pers Soc Psychol.* 2001;80(5):804-813.

Diener E, Chan MY. Happy people live longer: subjective well-being contributes to health and longevity. *Appl psychol. Health and Well-Being* 2011;3(1):1-43.

Demirci K, Mehmet A, Akpinara A. Relationship of smartphone use severity with sleep quality, depression, and anxiety in university students. *J Behav Addict.* 2015;4(2):85–9.

Eichstaedt JC. Schwartz HA, Kern ML, et al. Psychological language on twitter predicts county-level heart disease mortality. *Psychol Sci.* 2015;26(2):159-169.

Emmons RA, McCullough ME. Counting blessings versus burdens: an experimental investigation of gratitude and subjective well-being in daily life. *J Pers Soc Psychol.* 2003;84(2):377–389.

Eriksson S, Gard G. Physical exercise and depression. *Physical Therapy Reviews* 2011;16(4):261-268.

Ernst C, Olson AK, Pinel JP, et al. Antidepressant effects of exercise: evidence for an adult-neurogenesis hypothesis? *J Psychiat Neurosci.* 2006;31(2):83-92.

Ford ES, Bergmann MM, Kröger J, et al. Healthy living is the best revenge. Findings from the European Prospective Investigation into Cancer and Nutrition–Potsdam Study. *Arch Intern Med.* 2009;169(15):1355-1362.

Fredrickson BL. The broaden-and-build theory of positive emotions. *Philos Trans R Soc Lond B Biol Sci.* 2004;359(1449):1367-1378.

Fredrickson BL. Positive emotions broaden and build. *Advances in Experimental Soc Psychol.* 2013;47:1-53.

Fredrickson BL, Cohn MA, Coffey KA, et al. Open hearts build lives: Positive emotions, induced through loving-kindness meditation, build consequential personal resources. *J Pers Soc Psychol.* 2008;92:1045-1062.

Fredrickson BL, Grewen KM, Algoe SB, et al. Psychological well-being and the human conserved transcriptional response to adversity. *PLoS ONE.* 2015;10(3):e0121839.

Gardner MP, Wansink B, Kim J, et al. Better moods for better eating? How mood influences food choice. *J Consum Psychol.* 2014;24(3):320-335.

Gradisar M, Wolfson AR, Harvey AG, et al. The sleep and technology use of Americans: Findings from the National Sleep Foundation's 2011 Sleep in America Poll. *J Clin Sleep Med.* 2013;9(12):1291-1299.

Hansen CJ, Stevens LC, Coast R. Exercise duration and mood state: how much is enough to feel better? *Health Psychol.* 2001;20(4):267-275.

Hendriks T, Schotanus-Dijkstra M, Hassankhan A. et al. The efficacy of multi-component Positive Psychology Interventions: A systematic review and meta-analysis of Randomized Controlled Trials. *J Happiness Stud.* 2019:1-34.

Hirshkowitz M, Whiton K, Albert SM, et al. National Sleep Foundation's updated sleep duration recommendations: final report. *Sleep Health* 2015;1(4):233-243.

Huffman JC, Beale EE, Beach SR, et al. Design and baseline data from the Gratitude Research in Acute Coronary Events (GRACE) study. *Contemp Clin Trials* 2015;44:11-19.

Isgett SF, Kok BE, Baczkowski BM, et al. Influences of oxytocin and respiratory sinus arrythmia on emotions and social behavior in daily life. *Emotion* 2017;17:1156-1165.

Jacka FN. Association of Western and traditional diets with depression and anxiety in women. *Am J Psychiat.*2010;167:305-511.

Jacka FN. Kremer PJ, Berk M, et al. A prospective study of diet quality and mental health in adolescents. *PLoS One* 2011;6(9):e24805.

Jacka FN, O'Neil A, Opie R, et al. A randomized controlled trial of dietary improvement for adults with major depression (the 'SMILES' trial). *BMC Med.* 2017;15(1):23

Kaplan S. The restorative benefits of nature: Toward an integrative framework. *J Clin Psychiat.* 1995;66(10):1254–69.

Kim ES, Sun JK, Park N, et al. Purpose in life and reduced risk of myocardial infarction among older US adults with coronary heart disease: a two-year follow-up. *J Behav Med.* 2013;36(2):124-133.

Kim, ES, Strecher VJ, Ryff CD. Purpose in life and use of preventive health care services. *Proc Natl Acad Sci.* 2014;111(46):16331-16336.

Kok BE, Coffey KA, Cohn MA, et al. How positive emotions build physical health: perceived positive social connections account for the upward spiral between positive emotions and vagal tone. *Psychol Sci.* 2013;24:1123-1132.

Kok BE, Fredrickson BL. Upward spirals of the heart: Autonomic flexibility, as indexed by vagal tone, reciprocally and prospectively predicts positive emotions and social connectedness. *Biol Psychol.* 2010;85:432-436.

Kuo FE, Sullivan WC. Aggression and violence in the inner city: Effects of environment via mental fatigue. *Environ Behav.* 2001;33(4):543–71.

Kuo M. How might contact with nature promote human health? Promising mechanisms and a possible central pathway. *Front Psychol.* 2015, Aug 25. doi:10.3389/fpsyg.2015.01093.

Kyba CC, Kuester T, Sánchez de Miguel A, et al. Artificially lit surface of Earth at night increasing in radiance and extent. *Sci Adv.* 2017; 3:e1701528.

Lai JS, Hiles S, Bisquera A, et al. A systematic review and meta-analysis of dietary patterns and depression in community dwelling adults. *Am J Clin Nutr.* 2014;99(1):181-97.

Lam RW, Levitt AJ, Levitan RD, et al. Efficacy of bright light treatment, fluoxetine, and the combination in patients with nonseasonal Major Depressive Disorder: A Randomized Clinical Trial. *JAMA Psychiat.* 2016;73(1):56–63.

Lathia N, Sandstrom GM, Mascolo C, et al. Happier People Live More Active Lives: Using Smartphones to Link Happiness and Physical Activity. *PloS One* 2017;12(1):e0160589.

Lean ME, Leslie WS, Barnes AC, et al. Primary care-led weight management for remission of type 2 diabetes (DiRECT): an open-label, cluster-randomised trial. *Lancet* 2018; 391: 541–51.

Major B, Le Nguyen KD, Lundberg KB, et al. Well-being correlates of perceived positivity resonance: Evidence from trait and episode-level assessments. *Pers Soc Psychol Bull.* 2018:1631-1647.

Maller C, Townsend M, Pryor A, et al. Healthy nature healthy people: 'contact in nature' as an upstream health promotion intervention for populations. *Health Promot Int.* 2006;21(1):45-54.

Mammen G, Faulkner G. Physical activity and the prevention of depression: a systematic review of prospective studies. *Am J Prev Med.* 2013;45(5):649-657.

Mathur MB, Epel E, Kind S, et al. Perceived stress and telomere length: A systematic review, meta-analysis, and methodologic considerations for advancing the field. *Brain Behav Immun.* 2016;54:158-169.

McKercher C, Sanderson K, Schmidt MD, et al. Physical activity patterns and risk of depression in young adulthood: a 20-year cohort study since childhood. *Soc Psych Psych Epid.* 2014; 49(11):1823-34.

McMahon EA, Estes D. The effect of contact with natural environments on positive and negative affect: A meta-analysis. *J Posit Psychol.* 2015;(6):507-519.

Mikkelsen K, Stojanovska L, Polenakovic M, et al. Exercise and mental health. *Maturitas* 2017;106:48–56.

Mura G, Carta MG. Physical activity in depressed elderly: A systematic review. *Clinic Pract Epidemiol Mental Health* 2013;12(9):125-35.

Neckelmann D, Mykletun A, Dahl AA. Chronic insomnia as a risk factor for developing anxiety and depression. *Sleep* 2007;30(7):873-880.

Nelson-Coffey K, Fritz MM, Lyubomirsky S, et al. Kindness in the blood: A randomized controlled trial of the gene regulatory impact of prosocial behavior. *Psychoneuroendocr.* 2017;81:8-13.

Nutsford D, Perason AL, Kingham S. An ecological study investigating the association between access to urban green space and mental health. *Publ Health* 2013;127(11):1005-1011.

Ornish D, Brown SE, Scherwitz LW, et al. Can lifestyle changes reverse coronary heart disease? The Lifestyle Heart Trial. *Lancet* 1990;336:129-33.

Parletta N, Zarnowiecki D, Cho J, et al. A Mediterranean-style dietary intervention supplemented with fish oil improves diet quality and mental health in people with depression: A randomized controlled trial (HELFIMED). *Nutr Neurosci.* 2017:1-14.

Pearson DG, Craig T. The great outdoors? Exploring the mental health benefits of natural environments. *Front Psychol.* 2014;5(1178):1–4.

Redwine LS, Henry BS, Pung MA, et al. J Pilot randomized study of a gratitude journaling intervention on heart rate variability and inflammatory biomarkers in patients with stage B heart failure. *Psychosom Med.* 2016;78(6):667-76.

Rhodes RE, Kates KA. Can the affective response to exercise predict future motives and physical activity behavior? A systematic review of published evidence. *Ann Behav Med.* 2015;49(5):715-31.

Richards J, Jiang X, Kelly P, et al. Don't worry, be happy: cross-sectional associations between physical activity and happiness in 15 European countries. *BMC Public Health* 2015;15:53.

Riemann D, Voderholzer U. Primary insomnia: a risk factor to develop depression? *J Affect Disorders* 2003;76(1-3):255-259.

Rimer J, Dwan K, Lawlor DA, et al. Exercise for depression, *Cochrane Db Syst Rev.* 2012;11(7).

Sanchez-Villegas A, Toledo E, de Irata J, et al. Fast-food and commercial bakes goods consumption and the risk of depression. *Public Health Nutr.* 2012;15(3):424-432.

Sanchez-Villegas A. Dietary intake and the risk of depression: The SUN Project. *PLoS One.* 2011;6e16268.

Sandstrom GM, Dunn EW. Social interactions and well-being: The surprising power of weak ties. *Pers Soc Psychol B.* 2014;40:910-922.

Singh NA, Stavrinos TM, Scarbek Y, et al. A randomized controlled trial of high versus low intensity weight training versus general practitioner care for clinical depression in older adults. *J Gerontol.* 2005;60(6):768-776.

Stanton R, Reaburn P, Happell B. Is cardiovascular or resistance exercise better to treat patients with depression? A narrative review. *Issues Ment Health Nurs.* 2013;34(7):531-538.

Stickgold R. Sleep on it. *New Scientist* 2015;313(4):52-57.

Stothard ER, McHill AW, Depner CM, et al. Circadian entrainment to the natural light-dark cycle across seasons and the weekend. *Curr Biol.* 2016;27:1–6.

Tanihata T, Kanda H, Osaki Y, et al. Unhealthy lifestyle, poor mental health, and its correlation among adolescents: A nationwide cross-sectional survey. *Asia Pac J Public He.* 2015;27(2):NP1557-NP1565.

Tugade MM, Fredrickson BL, Barrett LF. Psychological resilience and positive emotional granularity: Examining the benefits of positive emotions on coping and health. *J Pers.* 2004; 72(6):1161-90.

Tuunainen A, Kripke DF, Endo T. Light therapy for non seasonal depression. *Cochrane Db Syst Rev.* 2010;2. Article No: CD004050.

Ulrich RS. View Through a window may influence recovery from surgery. *Science* 1984;224:420–1.

Valles-Colomer M, Falony G, Darzi Y, et al. The neuroactive potential of the human gut microbiota in quality of life and depression. *Nat Microbiol.* 2019;4:623–632.

Van Cappellen P, Rice EL, Catalino LI, et al. Positive affective processes underlie positive health behavior change. *Psychol Health* 2018;33:77-97.

Velten J, Lavalle KL, Scholten S, et al Lifestyle choices and mental health: a representative population survey. *BMC Psychol.* 2014;2:58.

Vyssoki B, Praschak-Rieder N, Sonneck G, et al. Effects of sunshine on suicide rates. *Compr Psychiat.* 2012;53:535–39.

Waugh CE, Fredrickson BL. Nice to know you: Positive emotions, self-other overlap, and complex understanding in the formation of a new relationship. *J Posit Psychol.* 2006;1:93-106.

White BA, Horwath CC, Conner TS. Many apples a day keep the blues away–daily experiences of negative and positive affect and food consumption in young adults. *Brit J Health Psychol.* 2013;18(4):782-798.

Yoo SS, Gujar N, Hu P, et al. The human emotional brain without sleep–a prefrontal amygdala disconnect. *Curr Biol.* 2007;17(20):877-878.

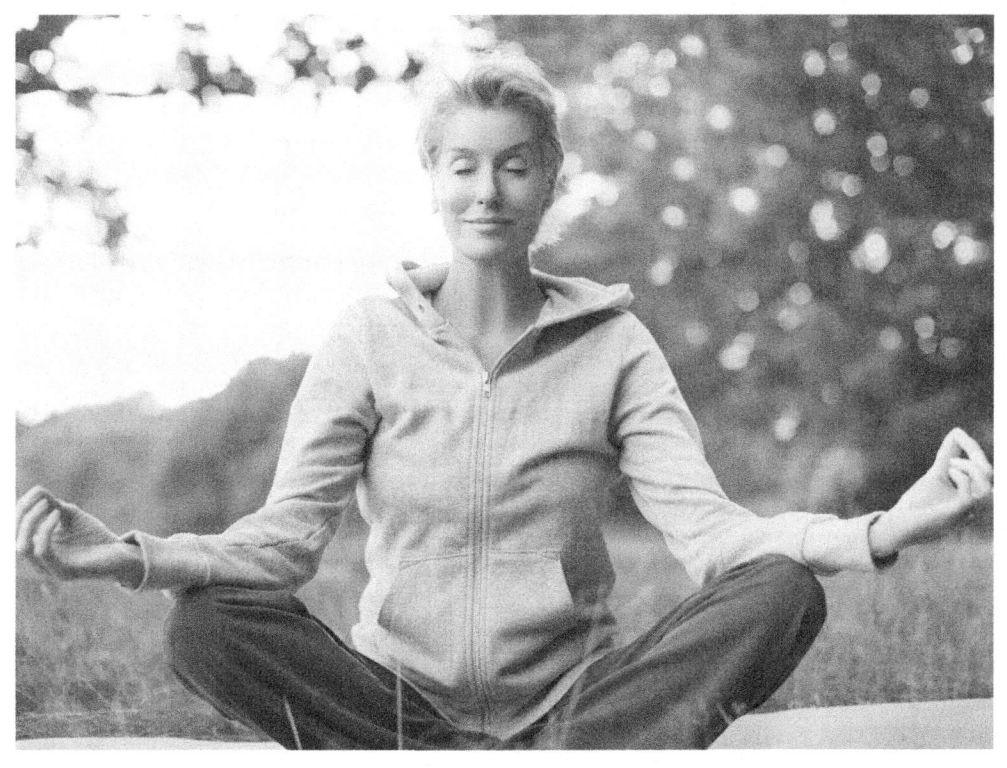

CHAPTER 3
Positive Psychology Interventions
Ingrid Edshteyn

Chapter Goal:
To describe key positive psychology interventions (PPIs) and their impact on emotional well-being and physical health, and provide guidance on how to prescribe these activities.

Chapter Highlights:
- Standard approaches to stress management focus on lessening negative emotions, but are not aimed specifically at boosting positive emotions for enhanced well-being.
- PPIs can be prescribed in health care to assist with stress management, improve mood, boost well-being, and facilitate health behavior change.
- Medical practitioners can prescribe activities, including activities that lead to a sense of flow (e.g. hobbies); gratitude practice; activities that are meaningful; acts of kindness; and social connection to enhance well-being.
- Religion and spirituality practices may also be essential for well-being among patients whose beliefs align with these practices.
- The impact of PPIs on affect, physiology, well-being, health outcomes, and longevity requires further research, but is an area that deserves attention from medical practitioners beyond the behavioral health sector.

Positive Psychology Interventions as Part of Health Care

PPIs enhance health beyond the traditional behavioral health approach. Standard behavioral health techniques focus on treating mental states diagnosed as clinical conditions that fit certain diagnostic criteria. Such techniques rely on removing the negative elements, such as anxiety, depression, post-traumatic stress or other negative psychological states, and reducing their burden. The focus is on moving away from the end of the spectrum described as mental illness toward improved mental and emotional functioning. The underlying assumption views negative and positive affect as different ends of the same continuum. However, a positive affect is not simply the absence of negative affect, and has potential benefits over and above removal of the negative affect (Pressman & Cohen 2005). We have an opportunity to enhance the positive, with resulting independent benefits to psychological health and function. This enhanced approach is the realm of PPIs in health care.

Medical practitioners aiming to promote mental health and emotional well-being may need to consider using techniques that can reduce the negative (mental illness treatment) or enhance the positive (PPIs). Some techniques may work in both domains. PPIs cultivate positive emotion and well-being not as supplementary, but as an essential and fundamental lifestyle medicine intervention that lays the groundwork for enabling healthy lifestyle choices and independent physiologic benefits. Such a refreshing treatment pathway offers solutions when working with difficult emotions and behaviors by strengthening new, positive conditioning patterns that counter harmful behavioral habits.

The additional benefit is that many of these strategies can be instructed and worked on independently by the client, not necessarily requiring a mental health professional for extended follow-up. The increasing availability of pragmatic PPIs reinforces a patient-centered locus of control and autonomy, reducing the reliance on what can be perceived as a difficult to access behavioral health system, especially for those with subclinical mental health conditions. Easily accessible and understandable PPI options are essential, and thankfully, numerous options are available.

A number of PP practices for cultivating well-being have been described for millennia. What can we learn from these traditions? They encourage a sense of ownership for one's own perspective and place value on the universal availability of a positive state of well-being by recognizing that emotional and mental health are not exclusively genetically determined nor fully culturally or socially conditioned. It is the historical understanding that emotional well-being is a skill of psychological function that can be developed and over which the individual has control, and therefore personal responsibility. Much like strength exercises train the physical body, training the mind will have an impact on one's psychological perspective, and can have emotional consequences. A positive state of well-being or happiness is, to a significant degree, a learned skill.

The field of PP has evaluated a number of potential interventions that can be applied across multiple settings and for a variety of needs. These resources are available to medical practitioners, even as the research builds and refines specific interventions for health care settings.

Key Positive Psychology Interventions That Can Be Prescribed

Some positive psychology interventions, such as mindfulness and meditation, can help induce feelings of calm and self-regulation, leading to a sense of well-being. Other interventions may boost positive affect with a sense of vigor and vitality. A combination of these interventions can lead to emotional well-being, life satisfaction, physical health and longevity. Hence, making recommendations for such interventions is fundamental to "lifestyle as medicine" counseling and promoting emotional well-being and physical health (Xu & Roberts 2010).

However, more research is needed regarding the types of interventions best suited for specific individuals across various cultural backgrounds and personality types (Chapter 7). Moreover, different interventions might be recommended for different aims. A number of PPIs, along with the salient research, are listed here as guidance so that practitioners can harness the research to date. As with most health and medical arenas, practitioners need to follow the release of new studies, lessons learned and recommendations for clinical practices based on translational research (Chapter 11) in this rapidly evolving field.

PPIs are being studied and implemented across psychology settings. Some are interventions that have evolved separately from positive psychology, but can contribute to boosting emotional well-being, such as the field of mindfulness and meditation. Many others correlate and align with the PERMA framework, outlined by Martin Seligman in his book, Flourish (2011), and described as the pillars of well-being. Seligman's five pillars of well-being include:

Positive emotion: intentionally engaging in experiences designed to elicit positive feelings

Engagement: becoming immersed in worthwhile pursuits that produce a sense of flow

Relationships: developing strong connections and relationships

Meaning: engaging in activities that fill one with a sense of purpose

Accomplishment: setting and striving for meaningful goals and embodying a growth mindset

Tables 1 through 8 offer sample prescriptions for individual PPIs. Another format is the FITT format (frequency, intensity, time and type of activity), similar to exercise prescriptions, as outlined by Beth Frates in *Lifestyle Medicine Handbook* (Frates et al 2019).

Mindfulness

Mindfulness is commonly defined as paying attention to present-moment experience, on purpose, with an attitude of acceptance or non-judgment (Kabat-Zinn 2009). Mindfulness is comprised of dimensions of self-regulation of attention on immediate experience and an orientation of non-judgmental openness to these arising experiences (Siegel 2007).

Most mindfulness-based interventions (MBIs) are derivatives of the paradigmatic mindfulness-based stress reduction program (MBSR). MBSR practices originate primarily from Buddhist and yogic meditative techniques. MBSR contains at least four main techniques, i.e., awareness of breath, awareness of body sensations, walking meditation, and mindful movement (Kabat-Zinn 1982). MBSR was initially developed to reduce subjective experiences of stress that result from chronic pain (Stahl & Goldstein 2010). Subsequently, it has been adapted into a variety of mindfulness-based practices, including those for clinical application, such as mindfulness based cognitive behavioral therapy (MBCBT) for general anxiety disorder (Evans et al 2008) and for prevention of relapse/recurrence in major depression (Teasdale et al 2000).

Mindfulness is often used as an umbrella term for a variety of practices, and individual MBIs can contain multiple styles of practice. Constituent practices such as gratitude, breath awareness, loving kindness and compassion are commonly prescribed. Other closely related meditation practices include loving-kindness meditation (LKM) (Zeng et al 2015) and compassion meditation (CM) exercises oriented toward enhancing unconditional, positive emotional states of kindness and compassion (Zeng et al 2017).

Mindfulness-based interventions (MBI) are effective in reducing a variety of mental health disorders including anxiety and depression, managing physical pain symptoms, supporting substance abuse recovery, reducing stress and promoting well-being (Creswell 2017; Engert et al 2017; Goldberg et al 2018).

Brief loving-kindness practice, designed to foster self-compassion, has been shown to produce higher positive affect and more positive explicit and implicit evaluations of self and others (Hutcherson et al 2008), and has also been shown to reduce depressive symptoms and increase positive emotions (Shahar et al 2015). One meta-analysis showed 1) medium effect sizes for LKM interventions on daily positive emotions in both wait-list controlled randomized control trials (RCTs) and non-RCT studies; and 2) small to large effect sizes for the ongoing practice of LKM on immediate positive emotions across different comparisons (Zeng et al 2015).

The benefits of meditation are well documented. But when recommending this practice, as with other interventions, practitioners need to keep in mind patient preferences, culture, spiritual/religious beliefs, and other individual differences. Negative outcomes, e.g., worsening depression and suicide, have been reported, especially among people with a history of substance abuse or psychiatric illness (Conner et al 2009). Meditation teachers and proponents may overstate the benefits and ignore the negative effects (Farias & Wikholmuel 2015). Research is examining the effects of different types of affect (a sense of calm versus a sense of vitality) on different outcomes, e.g., stress management versus improved health outcomes (Pressman et al 2019). Hence, staying up-to-date on this research and giving case-by-case clinical consideration is warranted.

Table 1. Sample Mindfulness Prescription

For:_____ Date:_____

℞ **Mindfulness practice, 1-3x daily. Dose: 1-30 minutes per session**
Go to www.mindful.org or similar website and explore different types of mindfulness practices. Find the mindfulness practice that fits for you.
Start slow and build duration/frequency at your pace.

REFILL: Unlimited _____, M.D.

Positive Psychology Interventions That Align with the PERMA Framework

Positive Emotions Derived from Gratitude Practice

Gratitude training significantly improved positive affect compared to breath awareness (d = 0.58) and loving-kindness led to significantly greater reductions in implicit negative affect compared to the control condition (d = 0.59) immediately after brief practice (Hirshberg et al 2018). Different styles of contemplative practice may produce different effects in the context of brief, introductory practice, and these differences may be heightened by stress (Hirshberg et al 2018). Gratitude as an intervention of counting blessings instead of burdens was shown to elicit heightened well-being across several outcome measures, with the effect on positive affect as the most robust finding (Emmons & McCullough 2003). Through the technique of practicing gratitude and thereby enhancing positive emotions, Emmons and McCullough (2003) posit gratitude builds psychological, social and spiritual resources, aligned with Fredrickson's broaden and build model to develop enduring personal resources (Fredrickson 1998).

Table 2. Sample Gratitude Prescription

For:_____ Date:_____

℞ Gratitude activity, 1-7x weekly. Dose: time to write 3 items
1. Keep a method for journaling at bedside.
2. PM: write down 3 things that happened that day for which you are grateful, or
3. AM: write down 3 things you are looking forward to that day.

REFILL: Unlimited _____, M.D.

Positive Emotions Boosted by Positive Activities

The techniques described above provide multiple variations of what could be considered generative positive activities, or practices that characterize naturally happy people, like expressing gratitude and practicing generosity. Based on the work of Lyubomirsky, such activities may serve as protective factors that reduce risk both directly and by impacting the underlying mechanisms of risk. Empirical evidence suggests positive activities promote well-being by boosting positive emotions, positive thoughts, positive behaviors, and need satisfaction (Lyubomirsky et al 2013). These positive activities impact the risk factors of rumination and loneliness and allow for adaptive coping from environmental stressors (Layous et al 2013). The value is that these activities may be learned at any stage in life and confer benefits for both physical and mental well-being.

Table 3: Sample Positive Activity Prescription

```
For:_____  Date:_____

℞   Random acts of kindness, 3 - 5x weekly. Dose: unlimited
    Each week, plan several random acts of kindness
    Something small like a compliment. Something large like organizing a fundraiser.
    Need inspiration? See randomactsofkindness.org.

REFILL: Unlimited _____, M.D.
```

Engagement and Flow

Based on the work of Mihaly Csikszentmihalyi, the concept of flow has potent application in the development of emotional well-being skill-building. The flow model suggests that the matched balance of perceived challenge and personal skills lead to optimal experience. Respondents in studies experienced the highest level of happiness while in flow, in other words, when the opportunities for actions in the surrounding environment matched the individual's abilities (Csikszentmihalyi & Csikszentmihalyi 1988). The process of continual growth and development by seeking out challenges in the environment and then developing the necessary skills to meet them may be a reliable way to bring about subjective well-being. The result is this sought-after "flow experience," the state felt during an activity that is going well, as if being carried effortlessly on a current. The defining feature is an intense experiential involvement in moment-to-moment activity, functioning at fullest capacity (Csikszentmihalyi & Larson 2014).

In this work that describes the conditions for experiencing flow, three are identified: 1) engaging in an activity that contains a clear set of goals that add direction and purpose (meaning) to behavior; 2) a balance between perceived challenges and perceived skills; and 3) the presence of clear and immediate feedback. The experience of happiness via completely absorbed attention may be related to the configuration of these components, set up to experience a positive state of flow. Enabling flow can be intentionally constructed with the three components necessary for its experience.

Table 4. Sample Flow Prescription

```
For:_____  Date:_____

℞   Flow activities, 1-3x weekly. Dose: unlimited
    Flow = being completely absorbed in an activity.
    What hobbies, games, work, or social activities are deeply absorbing for you?
    Find your "flow" activities and make time for them each week.

REFILL: Unlimited _____, M.D.
```

Relationships and Social Connection

A large-scale 9-month longitudinal study, the ReSource Project, found convincing evidence for psychosocial stress reduction after long-term mental training in a broadly accessible low-cost approach to acquiring psychosocial stress resilience. Short daily intersubjective practice may be a promising method for minimizing the incidence of chronic social stress–related disease (Engert et al 2017). Micro-moments of connectivity, as described in Chapter 2, have also been shown to have a positive health impact as a social connection intervention.

There is significant scientific evidence showing that social support and feeling connected can help people maintain a healthy body mass index, control blood sugars, improve cancer survival, decrease cardiovascular mortality, decrease depressive symptoms, mitigate posttraumatic stress disorder symptoms, and improve overall mental health. Counseling patients on increasing social connections, prescribing connection, and inquiring about quantity and quality of social interactions at routine visits is an integral component for prescribing this element of positive health (Martino et al 2016).

Table 5. Sample Social Connection Prescription

For:_____ Date:_____

℞ **Social connection activity, 1-3x weekly. Dose: unlimited**
Each week, plan time being with the people who bring you happiness or doing social activities you enjoy.
Not sure what those things are? Try something new.

REFILL: Unlimited _____, M.D.

Meaning and Purpose

Purpose in life is conceptualized as an individual's sense of directedness and sense of meaning in his or her life (Steger et al 2006). "Purpose in life" and "meaning in life" are often used interchangeably. The research shows that purpose in life has a positive influence on biological, psychological and behavioral outcomes and may even play an important role in protecting against heart disease in those at risk (Kim et al 2013). This outcome may be linked to greater self-care, as those with higher purpose had greater use of several preventive health care services and fewer nights spent hospitalized (Kim et al 2014). Higher levels of meaning have been shown to be clearly associated with better physical health, along with those behavioral factors that decrease the likelihood of negative health outcomes or increase those of positive health outcomes (Roepke et al 2014).

Table 6. Sample Meaning & Purpose Prescription

For:_____ Date:_____

℞ **Meaning & purpose activities, 1-3x weekly. Dose: unlimited**
Meaning & purpose = belonging to or serving something bigger than yourself.
What volunteer, work, social or spiritual activities fill you with meaning & purpose?
Identify what brings you meaning & purpose in life and make time for it each week.

REFILL: Unlimited _____, M.D.

Accomplishment

Feelings of accomplishment or achievement means using skills and effort to realize success (Seligman 2011). Individuals should be encouraged to pursue goals, both small and big, in their personal lives, as well as in their work lives. Self-directed goals that are achieved, providing a sense of accomplishment, contribute to flourishing and well-being.

Table 7: Sample Goal Setting Prescription

For:_____ Date:_____

℞ **Pursue a personal or career goal(s), 1-3x weekly. Dose: unlimited**
Successfully achieving goals gives a sense of accomplishment.
What goals can you set, either small or big, in one or more areas of your life?
Identify at least one goal that you can pursue confidently now.

REFILL: Unlimited _____, M.D.

Religion and Spirituality

Individuals use a variety of ways of understanding and dealing with life's challenges and finding meaning and purpose through religion and spirituality. These coping methods include benevolent religious reframing of negative situations, religious support, rites of passage, meditation and prayer, purification rituals, and conversion. Religious involvement entails multiple elements of the previously described positive interventions. Empirical studies have shown that these methods of religious coping are generally helpful to people and may even predict outcomes above and beyond the effects of secular coping methods (Falb et al 2014). Chida et al. (2009) found that religiosity and spirituality, measured primarily by involvement with a religious community, were correlated with decreased mortality rates among healthy groups, even after controlling for potentially confounding behaviors.

Religion may also provide benefit in the realm of self-control by providing a compass on moral behavior, with accompanying self-monitoring, behavioral management, emotional regulation, and prosocial action (Geyer & Baumeister 2005). In addition to these self-regulatory and social functions, religion has an anxiety-reducing outcome, particularly regarding mortality, as supported by a number of empirical studies (Soenke et al 2013). At the pinnacle of experience, religious and spiritual practices may also enable positive health via enabling a sense of transcendence, defined as "the capacity of individuals to stand outside of their immediate sense of time and place and to view life from a larger, more objective perspective … in which a person sees a fundamental unity underlying the diverse strivings of nature" (Piedmont 1999). Excitingly, these findings of spiritual transcendence, which can be measured by Piedmont's Spiritual Transcendence Scale, have been found to hold cross-culturally and are predictive of psychological outcomes such as positive affect, negative affect, and purpose in life, providing evidence of the universal nature of the transcendent aspect of spirituality (Falb & Pargament 2014).

Table 8. Sample Spirituality Prescription

For:_____ Date:_____

℞ **Time for prayer or contemplation, 1-7x weekly. Dose: 1 or more minute(s) daily**
Each week, plan time for prayer or contemplation.
Access the places or things that will support your practice (religious books or items, journals, place of worship, nature, etc.).

REFILL: Unlimited _____, M.D.

Summary

The research summarized here shows the potential for brief, yet regularly practiced PPIs, to cultivate the qualities of positive states and happiness. Feelings of calm and self-regulation, positive affect, a sense of vigor and vitality, and global life satisfaction are fundamental to "lifestyle as medicine" counseling, emotional well-being and health (Xu 2010). However, not all emotional states contribute equally. For example, calm feelings help address stress, but feelings of vigor might be more crucial to physical health and longevity. In this rapidly evolving field, researchers are teasing out which specific factors and interventions promote health and longevity (Pressman et al 2019). Medical practitioners can participate in the research, as outlined in Chapter 11, and need to be on the lookout for future study results and potential best practices.

References

Chida Y, Steptoe A, Powell LH. Religiosity/spirituality and morality: A systematic quantitative review. *Psychother Psychosom.* 2009;78:81–90.

Conner KR, Pinquart M, Gamble SA. Meta-analysis of depression and substance use among individuals with alcohol disorders. *J Subst Abuse Treat.* 2009;37(2):127-137.

Creswell JD. Mindfulness interventions. *Ann Rev Psychol.* 2017;68:491–516.

Csikszentmihalyi M, Csikszentmihalyi IS. Optimal Experience: *Psychological Studies of Flow in Consciousness.* New York: Cambridge University Press, 1988.

Csikszentmihalyi M. Flow: *The Psychology of Optimal Experience.* New York: Harper and Row, 1990.

Csikszentmihalyi M, Larson R. *Flow and the Foundations of Positive Psychology: The Collected Works of Mihaly Csikszentmihalyi.* New York City, NY: Springer, 2014.

Emmons RA, McCullough ME. Counting blessings versus burdens: Experimental studies of gratitude and subjective well-being. *J Pers Social Psychol.* 2003;84.2: 377-389.

Engert V, Ko BE, Papassotiriou I, et al. Specific reduction in cortisol stress reactivity after social but not attention-based mental training. *Sci Adv.* 2017;3(10):e1700495.

Evans S, Ferrando S, Findler M, et al. Mindfulness-based cognitive therapy for generalized anxiety disorder. *Anxiety Disord.* 2008;22(4):716-721.

Falb MD, Pargament KI. Religion, spirituality, and positive psychology: Strengthening well-being. *Perspectives on the Intersection of Multiculturalism and Posit Psychology,* Springer, Dordrecht. 2014,143-157.

Farias M, Wikholmuel C. *The Buddha Pill: Can Meditation Change You?* London: Watkins Publishing, 2015.

Fredrickson BL. What good are positive emotions? *Rev Gen Psychol.* 1998;2(3):300-319.

Frates B, Bonnet JP, Joseph R, Peterson JA. *Lifestyle Medicine Handbook, An Introduction to the Power of Healthy Habits.* Monterey, CA: Healthy Living, 2019.

Geyer AL, Baumeister RF. Religion, morality and self-control: Values, virtues, and vices. In Paloutzian RF, Park CL (Eds.), *Handbook of the Psychology of Religion and Spirituality.* New York: Guilford Press, 2005, pp. 412–432.

Goldberg SB, Tucker RP, Greene PA, et al. Mindfulness-based interventions for psychiatric disorders: A systematic review and meta-analysis. *Clin Psychol Rev.* 2018;59:52–60.

Hirshberg MJ. Goldberg SM, Schaefer SM, et al. Divergent effects of brief contemplative practices in response to an acute stressor: A randomized controlled trial of brief breath awareness, loving-kindness, gratitude or an attention control practice." *PloS One* 2018;13(12):e0207765.

Hutcherson CA, Seppala M, Gross JJ. Loving-kindness meditation increases social connectedness. *Emotion* 2008;8(5):720-724.

Kabat-Zinn J. An outpatient program in behavioral medicine for chronic pain patients based on the practice of mindfulness meditation: Theoretical considerations and preliminary results. *Gen Hosp Psychiat.* 1982;4(1):33–47.

Kabat-Zinn J. *Wherever you go, there you are: Mindfulness meditation in everyday life.* New York, NY: Hachette Books, 2009.

Kim ES, Strecher VJ, Ryff CD. Purpose in life and use of preventive health care services. *Proc Natl Acad Sci.* 2014;111(46):16331-16336.

Kim ES, Sun JK, Park N, et al. Purpose in life and reduced risk of myocardial infarction among older US adults with coronary heart disease: a two-year follow-up. *J Behav Med.* 2013;36(2), 124-133.

Layous K, Chancellor J, Lyubomirsky S. Positive activities as protective factors against mental; health conditions. *J Abnorm Psychol.* 2013;123:2-12.

Lyubomirsky S, Layous K. How do simple positive activities increase well-being? *Curr Dir Psychol Sci.* 2013;22(1):57-62.

Martino J, Pegg J, Frates EP. The connection prescription: using the power of social interactions and the deep desire for connectedness to empower health and wellness. *Am J Lifestyle Med.* 2016. Doi.oeg/10/1177/1559827615608788.

Piedmont RL. Does spirituality represent the sixth factor of personality? Spiritual transcendence and the five-factor model. *J Pers.* 1999;67, 985–1013.

Pressman S, Cohen S. Does positive affect influence health? *Psychol Bull.* 2005;131(6):925-971.

Pressman S, Jenkins BN, Moskowitz SD. Positive affect and health: What do we know and where next should we go? *Ann Rev Psychol.* 2019;70:627-650.

Garden M. Can Meditation Be Bad for You? *Humanist* Sept/Oct 2007.

Roepke AM, Jayawickreme E, Riffle OM. Meaning and health: a systemic review. *Appl Res Qual Life* 2014;9(4):1055-1079.

Seligman M. *Flourish: A Visionary New Understanding of Happiness and Well-being.* New York: Free Press, 2011.

Shahar B. Szepsenwol O, Zilcha-Mano S, et al. A wait-list randomized controlled trial of loving-kindness meditation programme for self-criticism. *Clin Psychol Psychother.* 2015;22(4):346-356.

Siegel DJ. *The Mindful Brain: Reflection and Attunement in the Cultivation of Well-Being.* New York, NY: WW Norton & Company, 2007.

Soenke M, Landua MJ, Greenberg J. Sacred armor: Religion's role as a buffer against the anxieties of life and the fear of death. In Pargament K (Ed.-in-Chief), Exline J, Jones J (Assoc. Eds.), *APA Handbooks in Psychology: APA Handbook of Psychology, Religion, and Spirituality: Vol. 1.* Washington, DC: American Psychological Association, 2013.

Stahl B, Goldstein E. *A Mindfulness-Based Stress Reduction Workbook.* Oakland, CA: New Harbinger Publications, 2010.

Steger MF, Frazier P, Oishi S, et al. The meaning in life questionnaire: Assessing presence of and search for meaning in life. *J Couns Psychol.* 2006;53:80–93.

Teasdale JD, Segal ZV, Williams JM, et al. Prevention of relapse/recurrence in major depression by mindfulness-based cognitive therapy. *J Consult Clin Psychol.* 2000;68(4):615.

Xu J, Roberts, RE. The power of positive emotions: It's a matter of life or death–subjective well-being and longevity over 28 years in a general population. *Health Psychol.* 2010;29:9-19.

Zeidan F, Johnson SK, Gordon NS, et al. Effects of Brief and Sham Mindfulness Meditation on Mood and Cardiovascular Variables. *J Altern Complem Med.* 2010;16(8):867–73.

Zeng A, Chiu CPK, Wang R, et al. The effect of loving kindness meditation on positive emotions: a meta-analytic review. *Front. Psychol.* 2015;6:1693.

Zeng X, Chio FHN, Oei TPS, et al. A systematic review of associations between amount of meditation practice and outcomes in interventions using the four immeasurables meditations. *Front Psychol.* 2017;8:141.

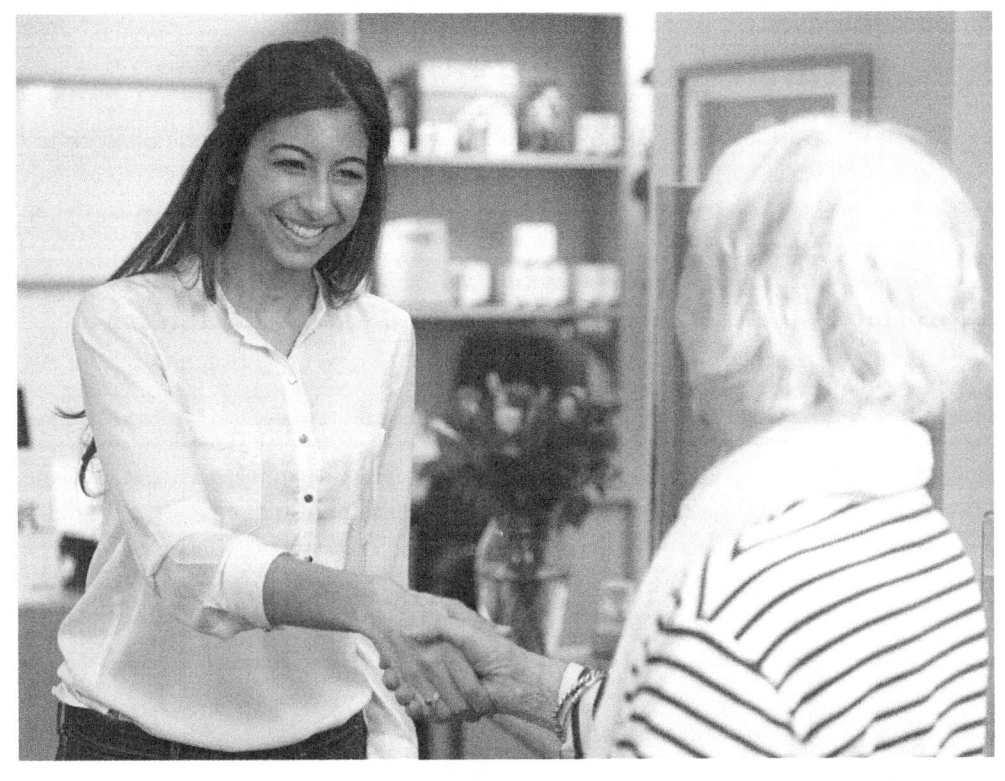

CHAPTER 4

Designing Health Care Practice to Harness Positive Psychology

Ingrid Edshteyn and Liana Lianov

Chapter Goal 1 (Assessment):
To guide medical practitioners on how to assess and monitor emotional well-being and positive psychology (PP) activities of patients, integrate PP into clinical encounters and prescribe positive psychology interventions (PPIs).

Chapter Highlights:
- Screening for anxiety, depression and stress, which are commonly encountered conditions in health care settings, can be conducted with brief tools such as the Patient Health Questionnaire (PHQ 4), the self-rating stress scale, and the Stress and Adversity Inventory (STRAIN).
- Medical practitioners (MPs) can routinely assess patients' level of life satisfaction with tools such as the Satisfaction with Life Scale (SWLS), as well as monitor the type and frequency of PP activities.

Chapter Goal 2 (Medical Practice Strategies):
To guide medical practitioners to design medical practices that address emotional well-being and leverage PPIs as part of a healthy lifestyle.

Chapter Highlights:
- PPIs, including vetted digital apps and programs, can be routinely prescribed to supplement mental health treatments and boost well-being of all patients.
- The 5 A's model and other behavior change techniques can be used during clinical encounters to assist the engagement of patients in PPIs.
- Medical practitioners can model PP-based constructs, such as optimism and gratitude, during clinical encounters.

Measuring Emotional Well-Being and Happiness in Health Care

The US Preventive Services Task Force (USPSTF) recommends screening for depression in adults (USPSTF 2016), but does not offer recommendations for anxiety or high stress screening, nor guidance for assessing the different dimensions of positive emotional states and well-being. At the present stage, the research literature on assessing and intervening to promote positive emotional states is not mature enough to make specific recommendations for standard health care practice. However, based on research in clinical and other psychology settings, a health care practice with the goal of promoting total well-being may consider offering positive emotion and emotional well-being screenings and assessments, along with depression, stress and anxiety screenings.

Assessing Depression, Anxiety and Stress

Two common mood disorders in outpatient settings are depression and anxiety, which frequently coexist. The Patient Health Questionnaire for Depression and Anxiety–the PHQ 4–is a valid ultra-brief tool for detecting both anxiety and depressive disorders (Kroenke & Spitzer 2009). Increasing PHQ-4 scores are strongly associated with functional impairment, disability days, and health care use (Kroenke & Spitzer 2009). The PHQ-4 is one way to spur a discussion about, and a prescription for, PPIs to reduce stress levels and anxiety and depression symptoms. MPs may need to initially prioritize these actions over lifestyle and treatment recommendations. Coping with negative emotions is more important for most people than sticking to a lifestyle-modification program. The perceived future benefits of lifestyle modification can be overwhelmed by feelings of deprivation in the immediate moment (Tice et al 2001).

Also, patients can be screened for high stress levels with a self-report of the level of stress on a scale of 1 to 10 (1 being the lowest level and 10 the highest level of stress). More in-depth screeners, such as the Perceived Stress Score (PSS) can be used to follow up with patients who report a level of 7 or greater (Cohen et al 1983; Lee 2012). In fact, questionnaires assessing perceived life stress, such as the PSS, are among the most frequently used instruments in stress research because they are inexpensive and easy to administer. Because of their low cost and ease of use, these scales have been extensively validated against many different health related outcomes, including physical and mental health complaints, brain structure and function, and biological aging. Scores of 20 or higher are generally considered indications of an unproductive level of stress. At the other end of the scale, scores that indicate low levels of stress–commonly, scores of 4 or lower–could be problematic since they signal an insufficient level of arousal.

Because frequent or chronic activation of the stress-related biological response is believed to be a key factor promoting disease, substantial interest has been generated in whether greater stress exposure across the life course is associated with poorer life-span health. An online system for systematically assessing lifetime stress exposure, called the Stress and Adversity Inventory (STRAIN), was designed to be an inexpensive, user-friendly, scalable, and reliable measurement tool that can be self- or interviewer-administered. The STRAIN has demonstrated good usability and acceptability; very good concurrent, discriminant, and predictive validity; and excellent test-retest reliability (Slavich & Shields 2018).

Assessing Life Satisfaction, Positive Emotions and Positive Activities

Despite lack of USPSTF recommendations, screening for negative states, anxiety and stress is increasingly common in health care, to supplement the recommended USPSTF depression screening. However, measurement of positive states, such as happiness and life satisfaction, is not generally part of routine intakes. The health coach community has been an early adopter of these assessments (Wellcoaches 2009). Interest in assessment of positive emotional states is rising in the broader health care community, especially due to the potential impact of positive states on health behaviors and in promoting improved outcomes (as described in Chapter 2).

However, because promoting positive health and prescribing PPIs are new goals for non-mental health clinical practices, consistent measures designed or adjusted for these settings have not yet been established. Some health care companies have added happiness to vital sign dashboards and care plans, but most measures have not been tested for routine use in medical clinics, and many of them are proprietary. MPs need to collaborate with PP and behavioral medicine researchers to develop happiness measures that are user-friendly for health care settings and relevant when monitoring patient progress. Chapter 11 summarizes key research areas for establishing this evidence base.

In the interim, ongoing PP research aims to sort out the most salient aspects of well-being that are protective of health outcomes, as well as the types of interventions that can make a difference in those outcomes. Psychologists are refining assessments that can be used in clinical psychology and counseling settings and virtual programs.

MPs can consider incorporating these assessments into clinic intakes and monitoring routines to get a picture of the patient's total well-being, spark a discussion with the patient about the important impact of emotional well-being on physical health and explore readiness to add or increase positive activities that have the potential to promote improved outcomes. In a busy medical practice, brief assessments that ask patients to rate their overall sense of well-being and life satisfaction may be most efficient. Assessing a patient in specific areas of well-being, such as the dimension of meaning and purpose, might be indicated when life satisfaction and other general well-being assessments are scored low. Examples include brief assessments of hope, flourishing, happiness, and satisfaction with life. Chapter 12 contains a more detailed list of assessments, and the Appendix C provides the items for a few key brief assessments.

One practical monitoring approach by medical practitioners can be to measure the frequency of their patients' PPIs rather than relying on self-reports of positive emotions which can be fleeting. A few questions about PPIs can be added to the routine intake, for example inquiring about gratitude and mindfulness practices, along with healthy eating and physical activity habits. Sample intake questions include:

- How often do you think about the good things in your life?
- How often do you take a few minutes to slow down and just focus on your breathing?
- How often do you engage in activities which are meaningful to you?
- How often do you savor your surroundings?
- How often do you feel joy and awe?
- How often do you share personal thoughts and feelings with someone?

Frequency options (daily, weekly, etc.) may be listed after each question.

Several other validated emotion and well-being measures can be considered for inclusion in well-being assessments. (See Appendix C for details.) These tools are often longer and might be more appropriate for health care settings engaged in research. A medical practice might integrate a variety of measures for certain populations, such as established patients who are working on positive activity action plans as part of treatment or who express interest in getting in-depth assessments and assistance.

Further testing and refinement are needed to identify and design measures for non-mental health care settings. Meanwhile, a few questions or short assessments that have been validated in psychology and mental health settings can be implemented in medical settings. These measures will remind both practitioners and patients about the element of emotional well-being as an essential part of health maintenance and treatment, spurring discussions that can inform total well-being action plans.

Facilitating Positive Psychology Interventions in Medical Encounters

Providers frequently follow a standard model or protocol for intervention when working with patients to change behaviors. One such model is the "5 A's", outlined in Table 1, historically used in tobacco cessation interventions, and also applicable to facilitating the use of PPI among patients.

Table 1: 5 A's Applied to PPIs

Ask – Identify and document the status of positive activities for every patient at every visit or consider inclusion of one or more of the assessments related to emotional well-being.

Advise – In a clear and personalized manner, describe the importance of positive activities in a "lifestyle as medicine" prescription.

Assess – Is the patient willing to consider one of the PPIs, especially if it may support improved health outcomes?

Assist – Provide in-office, affiliated health professional referral, online references or program referral for PPIs. Write a PPI as part of the clinical prescription.

Arrange – Ensure that you follow up on the status of the PPI at the next visit and keep a quantitative metric of progress, such as skill development or frequency of completion.

Adapted from reference: Glasgow et al 2006
https://www.uspreventiveservicestaskforce.org/Home/GetFileByID/440

What might it look like to use the "5 A's" in practice? While taking vital signs, the patient is "ask"-ed to rate the following on a scale of 1 strongly disagree to 5 strongly agree:
- I am satisfied with my life.
- I regularly do things that are meaningful to me and/or make me happy.
- Both questions provide insight into the patient's "positive health status," and the second in particular is excellent fodder for conversation about the types of meaningful or enjoyable activities the patient pursues and how often. Other verbal questions (similar to the intake questions suggested above) that can provoke useful conversation leading to PPI prescriptions include:
- How often do you think about the good things in your life?
- How often do you take a moment to stop, slow down, and take a few relaxing breaths?
- How often are you doing things you find meaningful, like volunteering, hobbies, or spending time with people you care about?
- How often do you just sit back and enjoy life, taking it all in?
- How often do you share personal thoughts and feelings with someone?

Such interactions are essential to facilitating action. Incorporating brief assessment and discussion of PPIs during routine intakes, diagnostic evaluations, behavior change coaching, and treatment planning can spur insights for developing a plan that addresses the patient's total well-being.

Even a brief conversation of this nature sets the stage for the next step, "advise", during which the practitioner and patient can discuss how the patient is already engaging in activities that promote well-being and the importance of doing so. Perhaps the patient–who is experiencing considerable stress related to his diagnosis of congestive heart failure–finds joy in bowling and card games with friends, but these activities occur infrequently. The next step, "assess," involves a brief discussion of whether he might bowl or play cards more often, or whether there are other activities the patient also enjoys that would help him feel better and lower his stress. As a result of this conversation, "assist" can include a PPI prescription for the patient, perhaps walking or working out at the local recreation center with a friend two or more times a week. (See Chapter 3 for additional PPI prescription examples.) At follow-up office visits, the frequency with which the patient engages in walking and working out, in addition to bowling and card games, can be asked and built upon or modified as needed.

For patients who find it challenging to identify activities that will promote emotional well-being, the Act-Belong-Commit model can be useful. This resource, created by a non-profit organization in Australia, Act-Belong-Commit and Mentally Healthy WA, is useful in exploring the activities, social connections, and engagements that provide meaning and purpose in life (Jalleh et al 2007). This community-based health promotion campaign encourages people to be proactive about their mental health and well-being and defines this process in 3 main steps:

Act: Keep active in as many ways as you can -physically, socially, mentally, and spiritually. In short..."Do Something!"

Belong: Keep connected to friends and family; get actively involved in groups of which you are a member; join in local community activities. That is…"Do Something with Someone!"

Commit: Commit to an interest or a cause; set goals to aim for; become a volunteer; learn a new skill; challenge yourself…"Do Something Meaningful!"

The organization provides a variety of ideas for taking action in each of the three areas, as well as a questionnaire that can guide discussion about the essential factors in the evolution of well-being and next steps for a patient to enhance well-being.

Additional Techniques to Facilitate Positive Psychology Interventions

In addition to the questions outlined above, the use of two techniques–powerful questions and affirmations–are key to facilitating insight and self-efficacy. Questions framed from the PP perspective include asking patients powerful questions to promote various forms of positive emotional states (adapted from Kubzansky et al 2018). For example:

- Optimism: "How do you think things will go with your health in the future?"
- Positive affect or life satisfaction: "How do you experience pleasure or satisfaction in your life?" "Are you satisfied with how your life has been going?"
- Gratitude: "What, if anything, do you have to feel grateful about in your life or with your health?"
- Personal strengths: "What are your best strengths and when have you applied them to your health?" "How might you apply them now?"

Moreover, offering patients examples of realistic, yet hopeful, affirmations to support PP elements during clinical encounters bolsters their self-efficacy and enhances their motivation for change. Examples include:

- Optimism: "I have managed many patients with this health condition before, and I have seen many of them do very well. I think you can too."
- Positive affect or life satisfaction: "A lot of research is finding connections between feeling happy or satisfied with your life, and your health. So I want to support you in taking time to do enjoyable and meaningful activities."
- Gratitude: "We were lucky to catch this problem when we did. I think there is a good chance that your health can remain strong if we work together."
- Personal strengths: "I have been so impressed with how you used your strength to overcome this life situation. You can use these same skills and strengths to be successful in taking care of your health."

Such statements, in turn, can be used to generate interest in PPI prescriptions. Examples are listed in Table 2. For additional detail regarding PPI prescriptions, see Chapter 3.

Table 2: Sample Positive Psychology Topics and Activities for Patients

Positive Psychology Attribute	Topic for Clinical Discussion	Patient Activity to Promote Positive Psychology Attribute
Optimism	Ask patients how they envision their optimal health future	Write out the vision of what optimal health could look like in 6 months to 1 year, and what steps could lead to this future
Positive affect	Ask patients to describe activities that bring joy or satisfaction (past and present)	Increase frequency of pleasant activities, notice the different positive emotions gained from pleasant activities
Using personal strengths	Ask patients to describe their character strengths or past successes, especially regarding health and leading a healthy lifestyle	Write about ways they have been successful in the past (especially regarding health) and what character strengths they used to succeed
Gratitude	Inquire about things patients are grateful for, especially regarding their health	Cultivate gratitude by keeping a gratitude journal or recalling three good things that happen (at least once a week)
Finding meaning	What brings meaning in a patient's life (health or otherwise)?	Record life goals and how well-being can be meaningful by bringing them closer to those goals

Changing Medical Practice to Adopt Positive Psychology Interventions

Mental/behavioral health settings have been using PPIs over the past couple decades. A review by Seligman noted that 51 PP techniques, delivered as additions to group or individual psychotherapy, were reported to produce increases in positive affect, with the strongest effect occurring when delivered in individual therapy settings to individuals strongly motivated to get well. They were also more effective when delivered over longer time periods (Seligman et al 2006).

Current research in medical populations shows that most applications of PP involve correlational studies with PPIs seldom applied. Hence well-tested, high quality PPIs with both healthy and medical populations, needed to build the PP-medical care evidence base, are in short supply (Macaskill 2016). Chapter 11 discusses how this research can be advanced. In the meantime, the medical community might need to consider adopting PPIs in medical practice based on research from behavioral health settings, in what can be thought of as "research-informed" practice. Leading PP researchers have shown that PPIs do indeed significantly enhance well-being and decrease depressive symptoms. "Clinicians should be encouraged to incorporate positive psychology techniques into their clinical work, particularly for treating clients who are depressed, relatively older, or highly motivated to improve" (Sin 2009, p.467). PP research findings also suggest that medical practitioners would do best to deliver PPIs as individual instead of group therapy and consistently over the long-term (Sin & Lyubomirsky 2009).

Given the substantive research on the health and well-being benefits of PPIs, it is up to medical practitioners to lead the movement of incorporating more PPIs into practice, especially for motivated patients, and evaluate emotional, mental, and physical health outcomes. The level of motivation for PPIs can be determined in assessments along with one or more emotional measures (described earlier in this chapter) as standard practice during initial encounters, and reassessed over time. Initially, referrals to behavioral health professionals and community resources can be made. As clinic processes are redesigned to accommodate PP strategies and patient demand for PPIs grows, PP resources can be built up with in-person or online individual or group offerings.

Sample Clinical Approach

To provide additional illustration of how medical practitioners can incorporate PPIs into clinical processes, consider the following example. The Act-Belong-Commit assessment was given and the patient scored low on the Commit scale, indicating the sense of meaning or purpose in their life would benefit from additional exploration. As a next step, the practitioner asked the patient to consider options for action. This step could be completed online outside of the clinic setting, with online or in-person follow-up.

Sample Patient Guidance

Make a list of the new positive activities you would like to learn or list some positive activities you already do. Set yourself a challenge or a goal to add or increase one of these activities. Take your time to think of a challenge that excites you and write it down as a goal. Make sure to include:
- *what you want to do*
- *when and where you will do it*
- *how long it will take*
- *what you need to achieve it*

If you feel your goal is too big, break it down into smaller daily, weekly, or monthly goals. Then set a start date.
1) Activity:
2) Challenge:
3) Start date:

As noted in the 5A's model description, critical to the patient's forward momentum is follow up from the medical practitioner at regular intervals to monitor progress, celebrate achievement, and refer to professionals in related fields when barriers or concerns arise that are beyond the scope of the practitioner's practice.

Partnering with Other Health Professionals

Working with other health professionals is one strategy for a busy medical practitioner to begin recommending PPIs and to supplement in-office resources.

Behavioral Health Professionals

In addition to developing brief in-office PPIs for patient encounters, partnering with behavioral health professionals can be valuable in achieving emotional well-being and health outcomes. These specialists working in the primary care, lifestyle medicine settings or other non-mental health settings benefit the clinic operational structure by offering dedicated time and continuity of sessions with patients to further explore, refine, and develop PP skills. Such partnerships can help distribute the resources across an interdisciplinary model and can coincide with the existing financial systems, where fees for services that include PP can be appropriately charged. While the medical practitioner may not be able to bill for PPIs, these interventions can be considered part of behavioral health services and would be aligned with current financial health care models.

A key to successful implementation of PPIs is for the clinician to approach this subject and set the stage for developing these skills, whether briefly on site, online, or in partnership with a behavioral health specialist. Counseling psychologists have been encouraged to claim PP as the logical extension of their humanistic roots and would also be natural partners for facilitating PPIs (Magyar-Moe et al 2015).

Health Coaches

While partnering with psychologists can be useful to advance PPIs, the clinic or health care system may not have psychologists readily available or insurance coverage may not be available. Medical practitioners can work with health coaches–who might be more accessible or provide coaching at lower out-of-pocket expense–to embed PPIs into the clinical practice model design. Referring to a health coach who utilizes PP in coaching techniques, or directly working with one on-site as part of an extension of clinical services, are strategies for emphasizing PPIs. Health coaches can encourage the regular exploration and skill-building required for the foundational development of PP skills and provide the context in which to nurture the growth of these skills. (See Chapter 6 on coaching.)

Partnering with Religious and Spiritual Counselors

For many individuals, their religious or spiritual community is a source of guidance and support. The positive health benefits of religious and spiritual practice, as described in Chapter 3, are numerous. It would be valuable to partner with counselors in religious and spiritual communities to help enable growth in the personal psychological realm. Religious and spiritual counselors can serve as trusted long-term contacts for patients, especially where clinical or health coaching options are limited.

Conducting In-Office Programs

Brief PPIs embedded within clinical care can be followed up with or enhanced with in-person or online programs that allow patients to explore PPIs. These programs can be completed by the patient on his own or with personalized coaching or therapy. The MBSR program discussed in Chapter 3 is one example of a stress management program that has been successfully integrated into clinical care. Many variations are possible that build from this kind of model, opening the door of opportunity to shift the landscape of how health is practiced in the clinical setting.

Referring to Community and Digital Resources

Small practices and other settings without in-house resources can consider providing recommendations for, or direct referrals to, meditation, relaxation, and PP resources in the community, e.g., churches, meditation and hobby groups or classes, mind-body programs, volunteer organizations, and senior centers. Supplementary resources for any health care setting, regardless of in-house programs, include online programs and smartphone apps from reputable vendors, such as the US Department of Veterans Affairs, the National Center for Telehealth & Technology, and others that have expert behavioral scientists as advisors. See Chapter 12 for additional examples. However, medical practitioners should note that most apps have not been well-tested to date.

Summary

Table 3 sums up these tips for medical practice redesign.

Table 3: Medical Practice Redesign to Incorporate Positive Psychology Approaches

Clinical Aim	Sample Tools and Actions
Measurement	
Assess stress, depression and anxiety	PHQ 4; stress scale 1 to 10; Perceived Stress Scale; STRAIN
Measure well-being status	Adult Hope Scale; Flourish Scale; Subjective Happiness Scale; Satisfaction with Life Scale
Measure positive activities	Happiness Skills Quiz
Measure specific elements of well-being, based on patient situation and interest	Meaning in Life Questionnaire's Mindful Attention and Awareness Scale
Clinical Encounter Techniques	
Discuss positive psychology elements for awareness, education, interest and patient status	Ask frequency of thinking about good things in one's life, being fully present, noticing feelings of joy and awe and sharing personal strengths with others
Coach positive activity behaviors	5 A's applied to positive activities; Act-Belong-Commit (do something, do something with someone, do something meaningful)
Affirm positive clinical observations	Discuss success of diagnostic and treatment status and progress; emphasize patient progress; highlight importance of positive activities; point out patient strengths
Prescribe PPIs	Add PPIs to a total healthy lifestyle treatment plan; include PPIs in action plans (when patient is ready) with details of what, when, how long, with whom, and a timeline; make sure these PPIs are varied over time, have an appropriate dose, and have an activity-person fit (See chapter 7 for details on personalizing PPI prescriptions)

Leveraging the Health Team and External Resources	
Partner with and refer to other professionals	Refer to behavioral health professionals, health coaches, religious and spiritual counselors
Refer to community resources	Refer to church groups, hobby and meditation classes and groups, senior centers
Recommend digital apps and programs	Digital resources are ever-evolving; partner with professionals who can provide lists of credible resources; prescribe them according to patient preferences

Medical Practice Re-Design for Positive Psychology Resources

Egger G, Binns A, Rossner S. *Lifestyle Medicine, Managing Diseases of Lifestyle in the 21st Century.* New York, New York: The McGraw-Hill Companies, 2011, chapters 13-16, p. 163-212.

Joseph S. (Ed), *Positive Psychology in Practice: Promoting Human Flourishing in Work, Health, Education and Everyday Life.* Hoboken, NJ: Wiley, 2015, parts III, V, VI.

Sin NL, Lyubomirsky S. Enhancing well-being and alleviating depressive symptoms with positive psychological interventions: A practice-friendly meta-analysis. *J Clin Psychol.* 2009;65:467-487.

Sinsky CA. Designing and regulating wisely: Removing barriers to joy in practice. *Ann Intern Med.* 2017;166990;677-678.

Example of Health System Addressing Total Well-Being:

https://www.va.gov/patientcenteredcare/features/expanding_the_VA_whole_health_system.asp

https://www.va.gov/patientcenteredcare/features/whole_health_the_veterans_experience.asp

Measurement Resources

Perceived Stress Scale (PSS): http://midss.org/content/perceived-scale-pss

Self Compassion Scale Short Form: http://self-compassion.org/wp-content/uploads/2015/02/ShortSCS.pdf

Stress and Adversity Inventory (STRAIN): https://www.uclastresslab.org/projects/strain-stress-and-adversity-inventory/

Other Resources

Act-Belong-Commit and Mentally Healthy WA (https://www.actbelongcommit.org.au)

References

Cohen S, Kamarack T. Mermelstein R. A global measure of perceived stress. *J Health Soc Behav.* 1983;24:386-386.

Coleman MT, Endsley S. Quality improvement: First steps. *Fam Prat Manag.* 1999;6(3):23-26.

Diener E, Emmons RA, Larsen RJ, et al. The Satisfaction with Life Scale. *J Pers Assess.* 1985;48(1):71-75.

Glasgow RE, Emont S, Miller DC. Assessing delivery of the five 'As' for patient-centered counseling. *Health Promot Int.* 2006;21(3):245-255.

Jalleh G, Donovan RJ, James R, et al. Process evaluation of the Act-Belong-Commit Mentally Healthy WA campaign: first 12 months. *Health Promot J Austr.* 2007;18(3):217-20.

Kroenke K, Spitzer RL. An ultra-brief screening scale for anxiety and depression: The PHQ-4. *Psychosomatics.* 50(6):613-621.

Kubzansky LD, Huffman JC, Boehm JK, et al. Positive psychological well-being and cardiovascular disease. JACC health promotion series. *J Am Coll Cardiol.* 2018;72(12):1382-1396.

Lee EH. Review of the psychometric evidence of the Perceived Stress Scale. *Asian Nur Res.* 2012;6(4):121-127.

Lyubomirsky S, Lepper H. A measure of subjective happiness: Preliminary reliability and construct validation. *Soc Indic Res.* 1999;46:137-155.

Macaskill A. Review of positive psychology applications in clinical medical populations. *Healthcare* 2016;4(3).

Magyar-Moe JL, Owens RL, Conoley CW. Positive psychological interventions in counseling: What every counseling psychologist should know. *Couns Psychol* 2015;43(4): 508-557.

Mason P, Rollnick S, Butler C. (Eds.). *Health Behavior Change.* London, UK: Churchill Livingstone, 2010.

Porges SW. Love: An emergent property of the mammalian autonomic nervous system." *Psychoneuroendocr.* 1998;23(8): 837-861.

Schotanus-Dijkstra M, Klooster PM ten, Drossaert CHC, et al. Validation of the Flourishing Scale in a sample of people with suboptimal levels of mental well-being. *BMC Psychol.* 2016;4:12.

Seligman MEP, Rashid T, Parks AC. *Am Psychol.* 2006;61(8):774-788.

Shields GS, Slavich GM. Lifetime stress exposure and health: A review of contemporary assessment methods and biological mechanisms. *Soc Personal Psychol Compass.* 2017;11(8).

Sin, NL, Lyubomirsky S. Enhancing well-being and alleviating depressive symptoms with positive psychological interventions: A practice-friendly meta-analysis. *J Clin Psychol.* 2009;65:467-487.

Slavich GM, Shields GS. Assessing lifetime stress exposure using the stress and adversity inventory for adults (Adult STRAIN): An overview and initial validation. *Psychosom Med.* 2018;80(1):17-27.

Thayer JF, Åhs F, Fredrikson M, et al. A meta-analysis of heart rate variability and neuroimaging studies: implications for heart rate variability as a marker of stress and health. *Neurosci. Biobehav.* 2012:36:747–756.

Tice DM, Bratslavsky E, Baumeister RF. Emotional distress regulation takes precedence over impulse control: If you feel bad, do it! *J Pers Soc Psychol.* 2001;80(1):53.

Tov W. Well-being concept and components. In E Diener, S Oishi, Tay L (Eds.). *Handbook of Well-Being.* Salt Lake City, UT: DEF Publishers, 2018.

USPSTF. Final recommendation, depression in adults screening. *JAMA.* 2016;315(4):380-7.

Wellcoaches. Clinical Assessments. In Moore M. Philadelphia, PA: *Coaching Psychology Manual,* Wolters-Kluwer, 2009.

Wellcoaches. Stress Management Guidelines. https://www.wellcoach.com/newsletters/images/Sress.Management.Guidelines.WC.8.05.pdf. Retrieved 4/17/19.

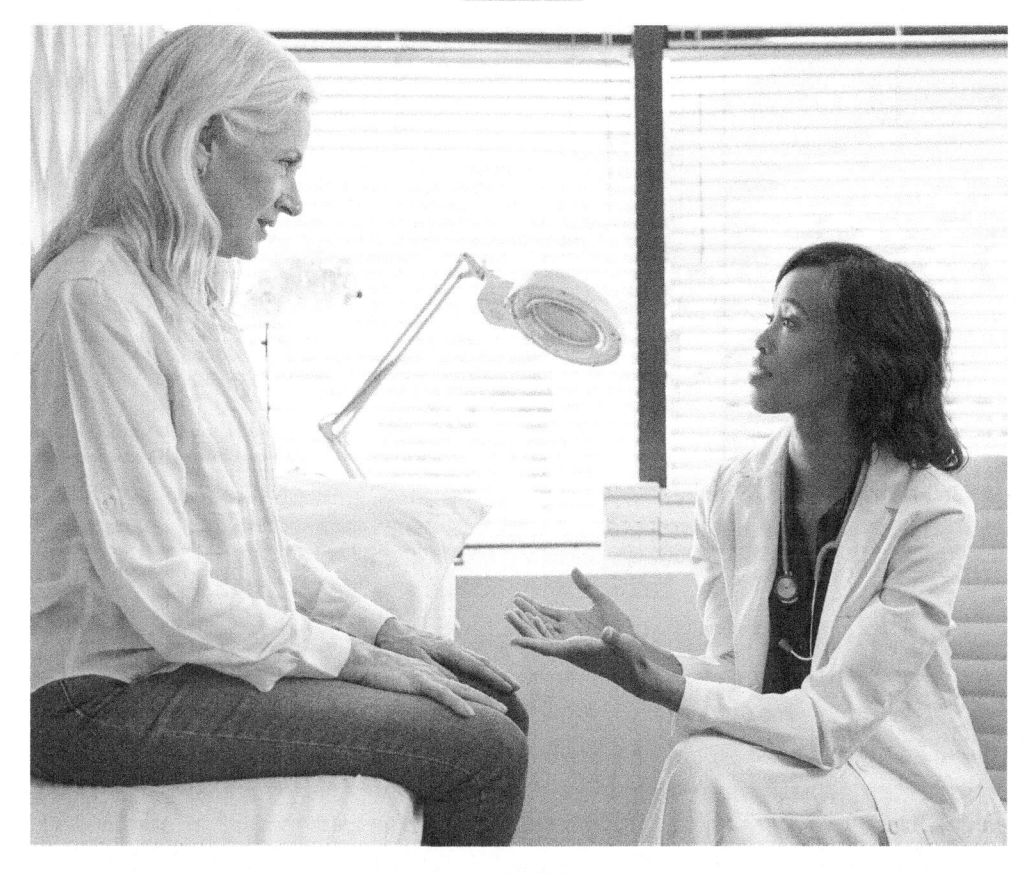

CHAPTER 5
Bringing the Positive Psychology Approach to the Exam Room
Anne Wallace

Chapter Goal:
To improve clinical interactions between medical practitioners and patients and to enhance health team member communication using positive psychology (PP) principles.

Chapter Highlights:
- Activities that boost positive emotions in patients not only have the potential to improve physical health and well-being, but also provider-patient interactions for satisfaction and results.
- Simple techniques during the clinical encounter can boost positive emotions, such as humor, attentive listening, smiling and focusing on what is good.
- Well established behavior change techniques, including motivational interviewing, can be enhanced with PP techniques.
- Medical practitioners can review their patient approach and clinical practices to determine which approaches for integrating PP principles would best align with their settings and patient populations.

Shifting Medical Practice to Support Total Well-Being

The notion that health is much more than the absence of disease is no longer novel. The World Health Organization has long defined health as, "a state of complete positive physical, mental and social well-being and not merely the absence of disease or infirmity" (World Health Organization 1946). In addition, the field of PP and its founder, Martin Seligman, have done much to advance thinking and research on the topic of positive health (Seligman 2008, 2012). Yet the practice of medicine, both inside and outside the exam room, remains largely focused on managing the symptoms of illness, pain and weakness.

This disparity stems from a variety of reasons, among them the lack of easily accessible, widely socialized practices in the medical community. The growing body of evidence and theory in the field of PP can provide a roadmap of techniques and strategies medical practitioners can begin to incorporate into routine patient encounters. Outlined below are some of the most accessible techniques that, with intention, practitioners can apply, even during brief encounters.

Building Positive Emotions

The benefits of positive emotions are well documented: they improve *physical health* (including fewer emergency room and hospital admissions), lower the incidence of drug and alcohol use, speed recovery from illness and injury, and are even associated with increased longevity (Fredrickson 2013; Lybuomirsky et al 2005). Positive emotions provide a buffer against *depressive symptoms* and help people recover from stress (Fredrickson 2013; Lybuomirsky et al 2005).

The relevance of positive emotions for medical practitioners extends beyond health impacts alone—they can be a powerful tool that informs the nature of patient-provider interactions. How so? Barbara Fredrickson's broaden and build theory of positive emotions provides a framework (Fredrickson 2001, 2013).

The broaden and build theory posits that people's experience of positive emotions (e.g., joy, gratitude, interest, pride, serenity) serves to expand their social, physical, and cognitive resources. Research demonstrates that when you are in a good mood, how you think is also positively impacted—you are more curious, more sociable, and more creative (Fredrickson 2013). You are better able to make complex decisions, becoming more thorough, efficient and flexible in your thinking (Boyatzis & Akriyou 2006). In fact, even small moments of "positively priming" one's emotions have been shown to directly translate into increased cognitive flexibility, speed, and accuracy. In one excellent and relevant example, researchers found that internists given a small gift of candy (but before eating it!) showed more flexible thinking and made accurate diagnoses of a patient with complex liver disease more quickly than those in a control group (Isen et al 1991).

Consider the following interaction as Chris's doctor walks into the exam room:

Doctor: *Chris, how are you? Oh, and in addition to hearing about how you're doing, I have a question for you... It's my question of the week: What happened in the past week that made you smile?*

Chris: (smiling) *I spent time with my grandchildren over the weekend. They are a bundle of energy – like little puppies rolling around! We went to the park and they just ran around from thing to thing, enjoying the sunshine and each other.*

Doctor: *Wow, that makes me smile just imagining it. Thanks for bringing me a little sunshine today! Now, how are you doing?*

Is this medical practitioner utilizing time wisely, asking patients a question of the week? If a goal of the session includes health behavior change and boosting well-being, the answer is a resounding "yes." To the extent that practitioners can cultivate positivity with patients, they are laying the foundation for patients to be at their best (Biswas-Diener 2012), and to think most creatively and expansively about what is possible. By introducing brief moments of positivity, (table 3) the practitioner is setting the stage for change.

Table 1: Tips for Building Positive Emotion in the Clinical Encounter

- Develop a rotating question of the week for kicking off patient visits. Make them positive questions that elicit information you'd appreciate knowing. Here are a few examples that may be useful to you:
    - What happened in the past week that made you smile?
    - What in your life brings you joy?
    - What's a favorite activity you've done recently?
    - What is one thing you are looking forward to in the coming week?
    - What's something fun you'd like to do in the near future?
- Use humor. Even corny jokes and bad puns that elicit eye rolls and groans evoke positive emotion. Laughter, after all, is the best medicine. What if humor is not your strength, but you'd like to give it a try? To make it easy, search online for "joke of the day" and have bad puns sent right to your inbox.
- At random intervals, bring a small token of appreciation to patients during office visits. A piece of fruit such as an apple makes a great option, particularly when combined with humor ("An apple a day keeps the doctor away…").
- Remember the basics of eye contact, smiling, and attentive listening. These are the building blocks of positivity resonance, enhancing social connection and positive emotion (Fredrickson 2013).
- And don't forget context. If patients have been kept waiting for long periods of time, are uncomfortable in a cold room (perhaps with just a dressing gown), or have had negative interactions/news in the office, a joke or uplifting question will feel out of sync. Instead, begin with acknowledgement of and empathy for their experience, and make right what you can. Knowing their trusted physician is in tune with their experience builds positivity resonance and lays the groundwork for forward positive movement.

Focusing on What Is Good

Let's pick up where we left off with Chris:

Doctor: *So, how are you doing? How are you feeling and how are you managing your diabetes?*

Chris: *Well, I guess I feel fine. My sugars have their ups and downs. I do sometimes struggle with desserts – I love them – and remembering to take my medicines.*

Doctor: *Thanks for sharing that with me. Let's first talk about your medications – how often do you remember to take them?*

Chris: *Um, maybe half the time? Some days are better than others.*

Doctor: *You're taking your medicine about half the time? Well that means you're halfway there! Let's talk about the good days. What's different about the days you remember to take your medicine?*

As Biswas-Diener notes in *Practicing Positive Psychology Coaching,* focusing on what is right and good, rather than on what is wrong, is a fundamental, philosophical view that is a prerequisite for all positive psychology interactions (Biswas-Diener 2012). Identifying success helps individuals make better short-term choices, regulate their behaviors, and gain the energy to move forward (Snyder et al 2002). While often easy to overlook, even the smallest successes are the building blocks for positive change. They provide clues about what existing healthy behaviors can be built upon, and calling attention to "the good" supports self-efficacy. Using powerful questions in the exam room (Table 2), medical practitioners can use current successes and positive health-related practices to support the shift from thought processes that inhibit health to thought processes that enhance health and, ultimately, enable individuals to flourish (Reynolds et al 2019).

Table 2: Tips for Focusing on What's Good

- Acknowledge and celebrate any success, no matter how small. Personal development is about embodying top moments more often than it is about changing the individual. And reflecting on what "is working" provides information medical practitioners can use to collaboratively identify an individual's next steps toward positive health behavior change.

- Ask powerful questions that enable patients to reflect on and gain insight regarding their successes. Questions that may facilitate insight include:
  - What is different about times you are able to…?
  - In those instances, how were you able to…?
  - What accounted for your success when you…?
  - Who supported you when you were able to…?
  - How do you feel on days when you're able to…?

- Ask patients to log activity related to the behavior of interest (e.g., healthy eating, medication adherence, exercise) for several days to a week. As they are logging information, ask patients to reflect on the strategies they used to help initiate and sustain the desired outcome. Perhaps they kept their medication, or their gym shoes, in plain sight? Perhaps they asked someone else to grocery shop for them? Intentionally implementing these strategies more broadly can lead to long-term health behavior change.

- Focus and build on the positive emotions that accompany success. Taking a moment to savor accomplishments builds self-efficacy and provides motivation for future action. We all enjoy a "pat on the back." Even better, support individuals in affirming themselves through regular self-reflection during journaling or behavior logs. Affirmation can include both congratulating themselves for what they've accomplished and how their body feels now that they've made the change. Chances are, by increasing healthy behaviors they'll also report feeling more energy, an improved outlook on life, feeling less stressed or other positive health-related benefits.

There is significant power in intentionally creating small moments of positive emotion and focus, such as those outlined above. Building in moments of positivity and highlighting what is working creates a powerful shift in the nature and tone of provider-patient interactions and sets the stage for empowering individuals toward positive health. Medical practitioners may bolster this work through use of additional PP coaching strategies during clinical encounters, such as those outlined in Chapter 6, or by prescribing PPIs such as those outlined in Chapter 4.

Integrating Positive Psychology Techniques into Motivational Interviewing

For many medical practitioners, questions arise about how to integrate PP techniques into their existing practices. (Some recommendations were discussed in Chapter 4.) Such questions are particularly true in relation to motivational interviewing (MI), a brief intervention approach commonly used in the medical field due to its effectiveness across a range of populations, settings and target problems (Hettema et al 2005), including weight management, heart health (control of cholesterol and blood pressure), and substance use/abuse (Rubak et al 2005).

MI is a process that helps people resolve their ambivalence and move toward healthy change. The medical practitioner creates an atmosphere conducive to change by following five general principles:
- Expressing empathy and demonstrating nonjudgmental understanding of the patient's perspective.
- Working to develop discrepancy by helping patients explore the gaps between their current behavior and the lives they would like to lead. Once this discrepancy is perceived, patients can begin to make the case for change.
- Avoiding argument by allowing the patient rather than the practitioner to present the reasons for change.
- Rolling with resistance by accepting the reality of ambivalence and inviting the patient to enter into the process of problem solving.
- Supporting self-efficacy, encouraging the patient's sense of the possibility of change.

Because both MI and PP coaching have their roots in Rogers' person-centered theory (Rubak et al 2005, International Coaching Federation), there exists much overlap between use of MI and PP strategies; they differ more in technique than in philosophical approach. Both MI and PP coaching emphasize an engaged and non-judgmental approach in which the practitioner listens actively and responds with empathy. Rather than providing expert advice, the practitioner affirms the individual, supports insight through powerful questions, and focuses on enhancing motivation and self-efficacy.

MI techniques have been integrated within PP coaching when individuals are reluctant to develop/work on goals (Reynolds et al 2019). Likewise, PP strategies can easily be woven into MI or other such techniques. For example, intentionally building positive resonance within patient-provider encounters sets the stage for more creative and flexible thinking as patients and practitioners work through ambivalence. Similarly, focusing on prior successes also supports overcoming ambivalence, enabling the patient to gain insight into ways they're already practicing the desired health outcome, whether weight management, enhanced exercise, or tobacco cessation. Chapter 5 provides more detail on how to use PP techniques in health coaching.

Engaging in Authentic Interactions and Relationships in the Medical Setting

Last, but not least, we include a couple of words on the medical practitioner and the fundamental need for authentic and trusting relationships. While this chapter focuses on the PP strategies that practitioners can use to elicit change in health-related behaviors, it is the quality of the patient-provider relationship that is paramount in the exam room, as it is in coaching (de Haan et al 2013). Similarly, and as noted by seminal figures in the world of MI, this approach is not just a set of techniques, but a way of "being with a client" (Miller & Rollnick 1991). In a very real sense, the practitioner–like a coach–is the most sensitive "tool" for creating change, insofar as she represents a bundle of basic, but vitally important, communication and interpersonal skills (Spence 2019). Or put another way, acquiring a new behavior requires interaction with trusted others in order to fully let go of old habits and adopt new ones (Boyatzis & Akriyou 2008). Ultimately, it is the power of authentic, trusted relationships in synergistic combination with personalized and relevant evidence-based practices that act as the catalyst in creating and sustaining health-related behavior change.

Summary

Building positive emotions during interactions with patients can benefit both patients and practitioners. Focusing on what is good, integrating PP techniques into motivational interviewing and engaging in authentic interactions with patients are a few strategies for bringing PP into the exam room.

References

Biswas-Diener R. *Practicing Positive Psychology Coaching: Assessment, Activities and Strategies for Success.* Hoboken, NJ: John Wiley & Sons, 2012.

Boyatzis RE. Leadership development from a complexity perspective. *Consult Psychol J: Pract Res.* 2008;60:298-313.

Boyatzis RE, Akrivou K. The ideal self as the driver of intentional change. *J Manage Develop.* 2006;25(7):624-642.

Fredrickson BL. The role of positive emotions in positive psychology: The broaden and build theory of positive emotions. *Am Psychol*. 2001;56(3):218–226.

Fredrickson BL. Positive emotions broaden and build. *Adv Exper Socl Psychol.* 2013;47:1-53.

de Haan E, Duckworth A, Birch D, et al. Executive coaching outcome research: The contribution of common factors such as relationship, personality match, and self-efficacy. *Consult Psychol J: Pract Res.* 2013;65(1):40.

Hettema J, Steele J, Miller WR. Motivational interviewing. *Ann Rev Clin Psycho*. 2005;1:91-111.

Miller WR, Rollnick SS. New York City, NY: The Guildford Press, *Motivational Interviewing*, 1991.

International Coaching Federation. https://coachfederation.org/core-competencies

Isen AM, Rosenzweig AS, Young MJ. The influence of positive affect on clinical problem solving. *Med Decis Making* 1991;11(3):221-227.

Lyubomirsky S, King L, Diener E. The benefits of frequent positive affect: Does happiness lead to success? *Psychol Bull.* 2005;131(6):803.

Reynolds R, Palmer S, Green S. Positive Psychology Coaching for Health and Wellbeing. In Green S, Palmer S. (Eds.). Abingdon, UK: Rutledge: *Positive Psychology Coaching in Practice,* 2019.

Rubak S, Sandbæk A, Lauritzen T, et al. Motivational interviewing: a systematic review and meta-analysis. *Br J Gen Pract.* 2005;55(513):305-12.

Snyder CR, Rand KL, Sigmon DR. Hope theory. Oxford, UK: Oxford University Press, *Handbook of Positive Psychology*, 2002, p. 257-276.

Seligman ME. Positive health. *Appl Psychol.* 2008;57:3-18.

Seligman ME. *Flourish: A Visionary New Understanding of Happiness and Well-being*. New York City, NY: Simon and Schuster, 2011.

Spence, GB. The stillness in growth: Mindfulness and its role in the coaching process. In Green, S, Palmer S. (Eds.). Abingdon, UR, Rutledge, *Positive Psychology Coaching in Practice*, 2019.

World Health Organization. Constitution, 1946.

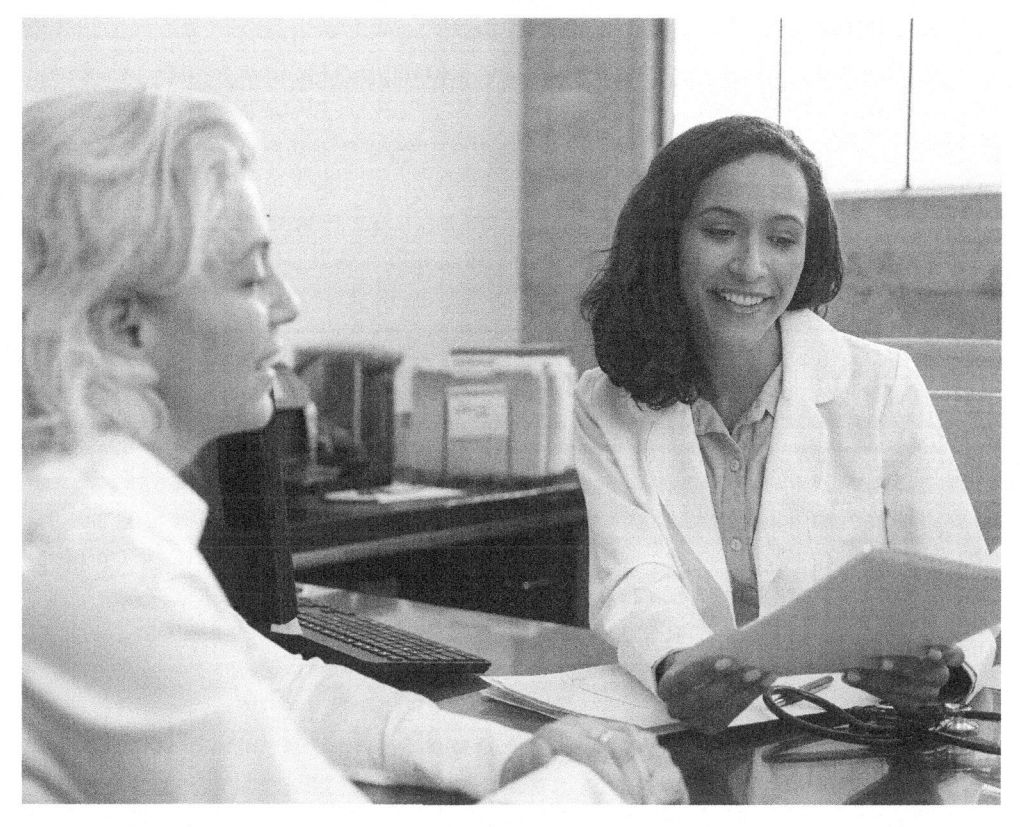

CHAPTER 6
Harnessing Positive Psychology Techniques In Health Behavior Change Coaching
Anne Wallace

Chapter Goal:
To review how positive psychology (PP) strategies can be implemented to improve behavior change coaching.

Chapter Highlights:
- Effective health and wellness coaching involves partnering with patients to facilitate self-discovery for advancing self-directed goals, offering education, serving as a source of accountability, and harnessing PP techniques.
- Prompting patients to envision a positive future is a key PP technique in coaching that helps propel action.
- Leveraging personal strengths is a PP technique essential to coaching and motivational interviewing, because it helps the individual tap into intrinsic motivation and is naturally satisfying.
- The PERMA model of flourishing can be used as a vehicle for connecting behaviors that are intrinsically satisfying with health-related behaviors.

Building Effective Coaching Practices

Health coaching is a comparatively young field of practice. Prior to 1990, coaching was generally limited to executive coaching used by CEOs and other top organizational leaders to enhance performance. In the 1990s, the popularity and prevalence of coaching expanded. With the dawn of the 21st century, coaching in a variety of domains–life coaching, health coaching, performance coaching among them–were increasingly becoming embedded as employer offerings to all employees, into health systems, and as a focus of wellness companies, not to mention the rise of "private practice" coaches "hanging up their shingles." Medical practitioners, especially those focused on healthy lifestyles as the root of treatment, need to, not only prescribe those behavior changes, but also do some coaching, even in settings where health coaches are available.

Despite coaching's relative fledgling status, many of its philosophical underpinnings, theories, and strategies date back decades and even centuries. While this provided the field some "legs" on which to stand, the early days of coaching felt a bit like the Wild West, where anything goes. The good news is, over recent decades, the evidence base has grown and standards of practice have been developed so that consensus has emerged regarding the coaching qualities, skills, tools and techniques that comprise the field of coaching for health and wellness.

The Essential Link between Positive Psychology and Health and Wellness Coaching

The International Consortium of Health and Wellness Coaches, founded in 2013, defines this branch of coaching as: "Health and wellness coaches partner with clients seeking self-directed, lasting changes, aligned with their values, which promote health and wellness and, thereby, enhance well-being. In the course of their work, health and wellness coaches display unconditional positive regard for their clients and a belief in their capacity for change; they honor that each client is an expert on his or her life, while ensuring that all interactions are respectful and non-judgmental" (International Consortium for Health and Wellness Coaching). This definition is based at least in part on a review of the coaching literature (Wolever et al 2013) which found that health and wellness coaching is fully or partially patient-centered (86% of articles), including patient-determined goals (71%), incorporating self-discovery and active learning processes versus more passive receipt of advice (63%), encouraging accountability for behaviors (86%), and providing some type of education to patients along with using coaching processes (91%).

At its root, coaching is a goal-driven activity. In most coaching engagements, the coaching process facilitates goal attainment and enhances well-being by helping individuals: 1) identify desired outcomes, 2) establish specific goals, 3) enhance motivation by building self-efficacy, 4) identify resources and formulate action plans, 5) monitor and evaluate progress, and 6) modify action plans. The monitor-evaluate-modification steps of this process constitute a simple cycle of self-regulated behavior that is key in creating intentional behavior change (Grant 2007).

Available research finds that health coaching is generally an effective strategy for promoting health behavior change (Hill et al 2016; Terry et al 2011), including improving nutrition, increasing physical activity, and improving adherence to medications (Alley et al

2016; Dennison et al 2014; Olsen 2010). Health coaching also has been shown to reduce health risks through mechanisms including decreases in body mass and weight loss (Allman-Farinelli et al 2016; Bennett et al 2010; Kivela et al 2014; Mao et al 2017), positive changes in blood pressure and lipid levels (Olsen & Nesbit 2010; Wayne et al 2015), and decreases in blood glucose and hemoglobin A1c (Newnham-Kanas et al 2009; Quinn et al 2011; Wayne et al 2015; Wolever et al 2010). In addition, research demonstrates the effectiveness of health and wellness coaching in improving the health status of individuals with chronic conditions, most notably through improved self-care regimen compliance (Hutchison & Breckon 2011).

Recent years have seen the incorporation of another young, dynamic field—positive psychology–into coaching. Marrying PP science with coaching allows for tremendous opportunity by integrating evidence-based techniques that enable flourishing into coaching's person-centered, goal-driven approaches and processes. As noted by Biswas-Diener (2012), PP science facilitates change within the coaching process by incorporating a positive focus, such as asking about what is right rather than wrong, capitalizing on the power of positive emotions, and incorporating the science of strengths. Of particular relevance to health and wellness coaching, Kaufman (2006) notes PP coaching suggests a language of strength and vision rather than weakness and pain. He notes that coaches with a PP orientation follow different "signposts and landmarks," looking for different information and cues when determining where to focus. Per Kaufman, while many clinicians follow "the trail of tears," those trained in PP coaching follow "the trail of dreams," identifying their vision of what they want and turning that into reality.

PP strategies can be used in brief medical encounters, as outlined in Chapter 5. Medical Practitioners looking to expand their work beyond short interactions with patients can also use a variety of PP coaching strategies outlined below, in support of lifestyle behavior change.

Envisioning a Positive Future

In addition to building positive emotion and giving attention to "the good," a key element of PP coaching is to connect the goal-setting process to a positive future vision. Research finds that positive images of the future pull us forward into action by fueling us with hope, putting us on the road to finding solutions, and helping us realize we have the power to make things happen (McQuaid et al 2019). Spending time taking stock of one's ideal self activates a range of positive emotions that serves to motivate people to make and sustain personal change (Boyatzis & Akriyou 2006). As such, a positive vision of the future – a vision of the type of person one aspires to be or the types of things one wishes to accomplish in life – is a fundamental driver of intentional personal change (Boyatzis & Akriyou 2006). Applied to health behavior, this shifts the focus from weight loss or tobacco cessation to a focus on how this change enhances the individual's life.

Consider the following interaction with Kerry:

Coach: *Kerry, we've talked about your goal of managing your diabetes. When you think about what it would be like to have your sugars in good control, what do you imagine? What would be different about how your feeling, and thinking? And what would it enable you to do that perhaps you can't do now?*

Kerry: *When I think about what I'd like to do differently, I go back to being with my grandkids. I'd have more energy when I'm with them. Maybe I'd even feel good enough to run around the park with them instead of watching from a bench! I want to be around for a long time and watch them grow up.*

Coach: *What a great picture of the future – I'd love to see you running around the park with your grandkids. What do you think about adding that to the goal of managing your diabetes? Maybe a goal along the lines of, "I will manage my diabetes so that I have more energy to play with my grandkids"?*

Kerry: *I think that sounds great.*

Coach: *Okay, I'm writing that out for you. How about you take this home and put it some place where you'll see it every day?*

Kerry: *I'll put it on my fridge – thanks!*

Traditional health-related goals such as, "I'll lose weight," "I'll quit smoking," or "I'll eat healthier," may be continual reminders of individual inadequacies and failures, of what one is not. Shifting the focus of a health-related goal to what one can become and what the change will allow one to do – to a very vivid and personal image of the future – helps people appreciate the future prior to realizing it, and provides the fuel to propel them forward, accelerating the change process. See Table 1 for tips.

Table 1: Tips for Envisioning a Positive Future

- Powerful questions are central to connecting health-related goals to a positive future vision. Asking people what they will be thinking, feeling, and doing differently invites a clear vision of the future, as does asking them to describe their future story, their image of what change "looks like." Questions that support uncovering a positive future include:
    - Imagine you've accomplished your goal. If you were to show me a video of you, what would I see? What are you doing… thinking? How are you feeling?
    - Think ahead to the future when you've… (accomplished your goal). What are you able to do that you couldn't do before you accomplished it?
    - What would making this change allow you to do? What would be different from what you can do or how you feel today?
- To support the change process, it's typically helpful to develop "implementation intentions" once a positive future vision has been identified. The positive future is "the what" while the implementation intentions are "the how" – the small steps that accumulate over time to create sustainable change. Helping individuals identify the next step that will support them in moving forward is a key component of actualizing the vision. Questions that support implementation intentions include:
    - What is a single, small thing you will change as a first step toward achieving your vision of the future?
    - Who can support you in achieving your vision?
    - What, if any, roadblocks will need to be overcome to…?
- Monitoring progress toward the individual's vision, in addition to progress toward their health-related goal, also enhances and sustains motivation. As people track their progress losing weight, regulating blood sugars, or taking medications, also ask them to log where they stand in keeping up with their grandchildren, the length of time they're able to garden, or how well they fit into that special outfit.

Leveraging Individual Strengths

Another pillar of PP science and coaching is the study and use of strengths in the service of well-being. Per one of the pioneers of PP coaching, Robert Biswas-Diener, "The idea that each individual possesses admirable attributes and that these are responsible for success and can be even better developed is essential to a positive psychology coaching practice" (Biswas-Diener 2012). People have a variety of strengths that arise in different contexts, from character strengths or positive personality traits such as perspective or self-regulation, to innate talents such as spatial reasoning or interpersonal abilities, to skills developed through practice (think of carpentry or surgery), and interests, such as painting, playing sports, and knitting (McQuaid et al 2019).

In collaboration with Seligman, PP researcher Chris Peterson determined 24 character strengths and divided them into six categories (Park & Peterson 2009):

1) Wisdom: creativity, curiosity, judgment, love of learning, perspective
2) Courage: bravery, perseverance, honesty, zest
3) Humanity: love, kindness, social intelligence
4) Teamwork: justice, fairness, leadership
5) Temperance: forgiveness, humility, prudence, self-regulation
6) Transcendence: appreciation of beauty and excellence, gratitude, hope, humor, spirituality

These researchers fashioned the Values-in-Action (VIA) survey to help individuals identify their top character strengths, as well as lesser strengths. Individuals can take the survey online at no charge at http://www.viacharacter.org/Survey/Account/Register. Other tips for identifying and using strengths are listed in Table 2.

Using personal strengths is energizing – people exercising their strengths become noticeably more engaged, enthusiastic, and communicative. Per Biswas-Diener (2012), using our strengths is like a favorable wind in our sails, propelling us forward more quickly and effectively than without their use. Individuals who use their strengths report lower levels of stress and depression, higher levels of positivity and vitality, and engage in more health behaviors (McQuaid et al 2019).

Let's check back in with Kerry:

Coach: *Kerry, we all know managing diabetes can be challenging. Tell me about a challenge in the past that you were successful in seeing through to the end. How did you make that happen?*

Kerry shares a time at work leading a large project with many different aspects to it, necessitating leadership, coordination, and persistence.

Coach: *It's impressive how you managed the complexity of that project and were able to navigate your way through to successfully completing it. Using your strengths and talents, like you did in that situation, can help make any challenging task easier. What qualities did you use during the project that you might also use to help manage your diabetes?*

When one learns to bring personal strengths to a challenge, it also helps that individual tap into intrinsic motivation, because using one's strengths is naturally satisfying. Consequently, using strengths helps improve one's performance and find more satisfaction in accomplishing tasks (Kaufman 2006). Particularly with challenging goals such as weight management or tobacco cessation, brainstorming and practicing how an individual's strengths can be applied to goal achievement eases effort and energizes action (Seligman et al 2005).

Table 2: Tips for Identifying and Using Strengths

- The first step is to identify an individual's strengths. Practitioners can do this is by spotting strengths in people as they are telling their "success story." A number of powerful questions can be used for this purpose, including:
  - Tell me about a past achievement. How did you make it happen?
  - Think back over the previous month. When were you at your best?
  - Among your family or friends, what are you "famous" for?
  - Tell me about a challenge you overcame. What qualities in you helped you do that?
  - What are you looking forward to in the near future?
  - What energizes you in the present?
- A more structured approach for identifying an individual's strengths is to use a strengths list (such as the example in Appendix D or ask individuals to take the Values in Action (VIA) survey.
- After identifying an individual's strengths, the next step is to determine how they can be used in the service of changing health-related behaviors. To manage their diabetes, one person may decide to use their strong organizational skills to schedule diabetes-related tasks on their calendar. Another might use relationship skills to talk through their challenges with trusted others and ask for accountability in making needed changes. A third might use the strength of insight to think through current barriers and problem-solve solutions.
- Key to talking with people about identifying and using their strengths is to explain the benefits that accrue from using strengths – enhanced motivation, improved performance, and greater satisfaction with the process. With the understanding that strengths use puts the proverbial "wind in their sails," people are more likely to engage in continued, intentional use of strengths in the service of health behavior change.

Connecting Health Behaviors to Intrinsically Satisfying Activities

Of course, the field of PP research and coaching was not initially concerned with health behaviors, but more broadly focused on promoting flourishing for optimal human functioning. As noted in Chapter 3, seminal to the notion of flourishing has been the PERMA framework, outlined by Martin Seligman in his book, *Flourish* (Seligman 2011), which he described as the pillars to well-being. To recap, those five pillars include:

Positive emotion: intentionally engaging in experiences designed to elicit positive feelings

Engagement: becoming immersed in worthwhile pursuits that produce a sense of flow

Relationships: developing strong connections and relationships

Meaning: engaging in activities that fill one with a sense of purpose

Accomplishment: setting and striving for meaningful goals and embodying a growth mindset

While traditionally the PERMA model has been used as a framework for promoting flourishing (Falecki et al 2019), it can also be used as a vehicle for connecting behaviors that are intrinsically satisfying with health-related behaviors, which often do not carry the same internal motivational attributes. Evidence is mounting that positive emotions in particular have this effect; when people experience positive emotions during health-related behaviors, there are motivational and behavioral consequences. Barbara Fredrickson's upward spiral of lifestyle change research finds that people who experience positive emotions while engaging in health-related behaviors become more flexible and creative in their behavioral choices in a way that activates and supports engagement in future health behaviors (Fredrickson 2013). As described in Chapter 2, this upward spiral of motivation and health behaviors is consequential for long-term behavioral maintenance (Fredrickson 2013; Van Cappellen et al 2018). Kaufman's connection of the intrinsic motivation that arises when engagement and purpose are present in a task supports this notion (Kaufman 2007). When meaning or flow isn't automatically present in a task, a key to future behavior change lies in helping individuals find those aspects of the task that are intrinsically rewarding.

How might Kerry use PERMA to support management of their diabetes?
Coach: *Kerry, I know many aspects of caring for diabetes are not fun. I also know that when people connect activities they don't enjoy with things they find satisfying, it makes it easier to "get it done." For example, people who don't like exercise (but know it's good for them) make it more enjoyable by doing it with a friend, or more interesting by challenging themselves. I'm wondering whether there's a way to help you remember to take your medication by connecting it to something you find satisfying. As options, you might create a challenge for yourself, connect taking your medicine to something meaningful to you, or perhaps find a "medication buddy." What sounds like something you might try?*
Kerry: *You know, I'm thinking about my grandkids. They are my main motivation for being healthy. I think if I put a picture of my grandkids right on the kitchen counter where I can see it while I'm making meals, I'll have a reminder about why healthy meals with lots of vegetables are important to me.... and actually eat them.*

All elements of PERMA can be used in the service of promoting and sustaining health behavior change. Moreover, the pillars of PERMA are not independent–they are interrelated and interwoven (Falecki et al 2019). Any one activity may incorporate multiple aspects of PERMA. In the world of PP coaching, the more pillars of PERMA individuals connect to health-related behaviors, the better (Table 3).

Table 3: Tips for Using PERMA

- Using PERMA starts with an honest conversation about the extent to which different health-related behaviors are intrinsically satisfying and motivating for an individual. For example, someone who is motivated to eat healthily does not need PERMA in the same way as the person attached to a diet of burgers and fries.
- A visual or handout is frequently helpful when explaining PERMA to people. Feel free to use the visual in Appendix A if it applies to your work.
- At times, a health behavior's connection to PERMA is obvious. The advice to "find a form of exercise you enjoy" is far from novel. When exercise or other health-related behaviors are not intrinsically enjoyable, intentionally connecting them to other enjoyable activities–such as strength training while listening to a favorite playlist or walking on the treadmill while enjoying a television show–suddenly makes them much more appealing.
- Some pillars of PERMA, such as engagement, can be challenging for many individuals to connect to health-related behaviors. However, engagement is a wonderful pathway to self-care and stress reduction. Activities that promote flow re-energize and renew the body and mind in ways that many more widely used "de-stressing" techniques such as media and social media do not.
- As mentioned above, any one health behavior can activate multiple domains of PERMA. Think, for example, of running clubs. Runners show up to connect with like-minded individuals (enhancing R), engage in a process that promotes flow (activating E) and set goals to complete a race or better their time (engage in A). With PERMA, more is better. Helping people connect multiple aspects of PERMA to health behaviors synergistically supports and enhances the motivation for change.

Summary

PP coaching strategies hold great promise for medical practitioners working to support individuals in moving toward well-being, identifying their personal and unique vision of positive health, and determining how they will use their internal and external resources and strengths in achieving that vision. Use of individual strengths and the elements PERMA support forward movement, enhanced motivation, energy and ease with which individuals' goals can be accomplished. At root are the core beliefs that change occurs within authentic and trusted relationships, and individuals are experts with regard to their personal needs and lifestyles who have the capacity for change and desire for growth. The work of the medical practitioner is to facilitate and guide positive change within individuals, empowering their journey to realize their "best self" and "best life."

References

Alley S, Jennings C, Plotnikoff RC, et al. Web-based video-coaching to assist an automated computer-tailored physical activity intervention for inactive adults: a randomized controlled trial. *J Med Internet Res.* 2016;18(8):e223.

Allman-Farinelli M, Partridge SR, McGeechan K, et al. A mobile health lifestyle program for prevention of weight gain in young adults (TXT2BFiT): nine-month outcomes of a randomized controlled trial. *JMIR Mhealth Uhealth* 2016;4(2):e78.

Bennett GG, Herring SJ, Puleo E, et al. Web-based weight loss in primary care: a randomized controlled trial. *Obesity* (Silver Spring) 2010;18(2):308-313.

Biswas-Diener R. *Practicing Positive Psychology Coaching: Assessment, Activities and Strategies for Success.* Hoboken, NJ: John Wiley & Sons, 2012.

Boyatzis RE, Akrivou K. The ideal self as the driver of intentional change. *J Manage Development* 2006;25(7):624-642.

Dennison L, Morrison L, Lloyd S, et al. Does brief telephone support improve engagement with a web-based weight management intervention? Randomized controlled trial. *J Med Internet Res.* 2014;16(3):e95.

Falecki D, Leach C, Green S. PERMA-powered coaching: Building foundations for a flourishing life. In Green S, Palmer S. (Eds.). *Positive Psychology Coaching in Practice.* Oxford, UK: Routledge, 2019.

Fredrickson BL. Positive emotions broaden and build. Advances in experimental social psychology. *Acad Press* 2013;47:1-53.

Grant AM, Cavanagh MJ. Evidence-based coaching: Flourishing or languishing? *Australian Psychol.* 2007;42(4):239-254.

Hill B, Richardson B, Skouteris H. Do we know how to design effective health coaching interventions: a systematic review of the state of the literature. *Am J Health Promot.* 2015;29(5):e158-e168.

Hutchison AJ, Breckon JD. A review of telephone coaching services for people with long-term conditions. *J Telemed Telecare* 2011;17(8):451-458.

Kivelä K, Elo S, Kyngäs H, et al. The effects of health coaching on adult patients with chronic diseases: a systematic review. Patient Educ Couns. 2014;97(2):147-157.

Kaufman C. Positive Psychology: The science at the heart of coaching. In Stober D, Grant A. (Eds.). *Evidence-Based Coaching: Putting Best Practices to Work for Your Clients,* Hoboken, NJ: John Wiley & Sons, 2006.

Mao AY, Chen C, Magana C, et al. A mobile phone-based health coaching intervention for weight loss and blood pressure reduction in a national payer population: a retrospective study. *JMIR Mhealth Uhealth* 2017;5(6):e80.

McQuaid M, Niemiec R, and Doman F. A character strengths-based approach to positive psychology. Positive Psychology Coaching for Health and Wellbeing. In Green S, Palmer S. (Eds.). Oxford, UK: Rutledge, *Positive Psychology Coaching in Practice,* 2019.

National Board of Health and Wellness Coaching: https://nbhwc.org

Newnham-Kanas C, Gorczynski P, Morrow D, et al. Annotated bibliography of life coaching and health research. *Int J Evid Based Coach Mentor.* 2009;7(1):39-103.

Olsen JM, Nesbitt BJ. Health coaching to improve healthy lifestyle behaviors: an integrative review. *Am J Health Promot.* 2010;25(1):e1-e12.

Park N, Peterson C. Character strengths: Research and practice. *J Coll Character* 2009;10(4).

Quinn CC, Shardell MD, Terrin ML, et al. Cluster-randomized trial of a mobile phone personalized behavioral intervention for blood glucose control. *Diabetes Care* 2011;34(9):1934-1942.

Seligman MEP. *Flourish: A Visionary New Understanding of Happiness and Well-Being.* New York City, NY: Simon and Schuster, 2011.

Seligman ME, Steen TA, Park N, et al. Positive psychology progress: empirical validation of interventions. *Am Psychologist* 2005;60(5):410.

Terry PE, Seaverson EL, Grossmeier J, Anderson DR. Effectiveness of a worksite telephone-based weight management program. *Am J Health Promot.* 2011;25(3):186-189.

Van Cappellen P, Rice EL, Catalino LI, et al. Positive affective processes underlie positive health behavior change. *Psychol Health* 2018;2;33(1):77-97.

Wayne N, Perez DF, Kaplan DM, et al. Health coaching reduces HbA1c in type 2 diabetic patients from a lower-socioeconomic status community: a randomized controlled trial. *J Med Internet Res.* 2015;17(10):e224.

Wolever RQ, Dreusicke M, Fikkan J, et al. Integrative health coaching for patients with type 2 diabetes: a randomized clinical trial. *Diabetes Educ.* 2010;36(4):629-39.

Wolever RQ, Simmons LA, Sforzo GA, et al. A systematic review of the literature on health and wellness coaching. *Glob. Adv. Health Med.* 2013;4:38-57.

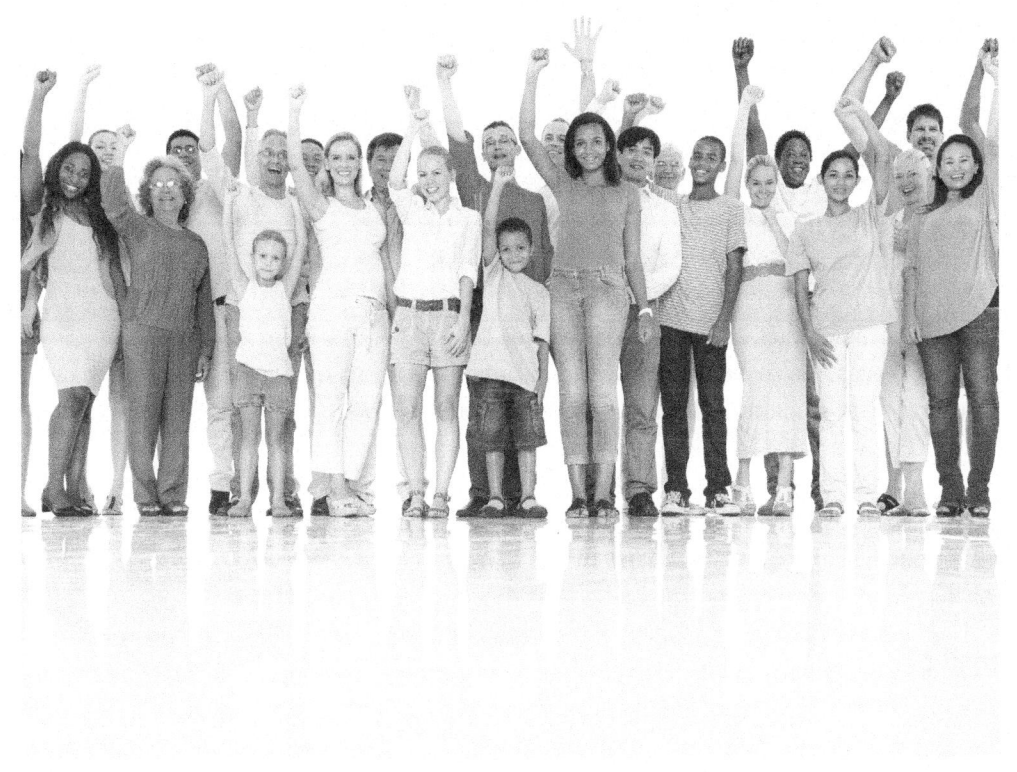

CHAPTER 7
Personalizing Positive Psychology Interventions
Liana Lianov

Chapter Goal:
To provide guidance on how medical practitioners (MPs) can recommend personalized positive psychology interventions (PPIs) that align with each patient's culture, personal preferences and personality.

Chapter Highlights:
- Research shows that individuals can engage in intentional positive activities to boost and sustain happiness levels. Such activities can be prescribed as PPIs.
- A wide range of PPIs have been applied with varying success. To increase the potential for success, these activities should have a good fit with the individual's culture, personality, and preferences.
- One key strategy for successfully sustaining positive emotions derived from PPIs is to vary the activities over time and avoid habituation.
- Timing and "dosage" of the positive activities need to be considered when prescribing them.
- MPs can recommend that patients conduct personality self-assessments to guide the selection of positive activities, with the potential for greater sustainability and impact on well-being.

Intentional Positive Activities

A number of studies show that happiness levels can be intentionally increased through a variety of activities (Sin & Lyubomirsky 2009). The negative argument against offering these interventions is that the happiness levels are not sustained, because individuals revert to a genetically determined set-point. A number of sources cite 50% as the percentage of happiness across populations that is influenced by genetics (Braungart et al 1992; Roysamb et al 2002). The actual percentage is not known, with a wide range being cited, even up to 80% (Lykken & Tellegen 1996). Even though this information can be discouraging, it's important to keep in mind that such data are relevant to populations, not specific individuals. Moreover, individuals can minimize or counter the effects of their genetics through intentional positive activities. Research shows that people encouraged to do positive activities can increase their well-being (Sin & Lyubomirsky 2009).

In fact, some researchers have found that happiness due to unexpected positive circumstances is not as well maintained as happiness due to intentional activities (Sheldon 2006). A growing literature suggests small sustainable boosts are possible through intentional activities (Layous et al 2015). Even if happiness levels are not sustainable in some individuals for the long term, short term boosts of positive emotion can have physiologic benefits, such as frequent moments of micro-connectivity that increase heart rate variability (HRV) (Kok & Fredrickson 2010; Van Cappellen et al 2018).

Because increasing happiness through intentional positive activities has been associated with better health, among other benefits (Fredrickson 2008), medical practitioners can consider adding such activities to the total well-being prescription. They can "prescribe" PPIs and encourage patients to engage in these activities along with other healthy lifestyle activities.

The Range of Positive Psychology Interventions

The spectrum of PPIs is wide ranging from brief gratitude exercises to more complex "flow" hobbies that might require special equipment and a specific location. Gratitude, optimism and prosocial behaviors are among the most studied and most consistently associated with reports of greater happiness (Heferon 2015). Hendriks et al. (2018) identified over 15 types of interventions that have been studied and shown to improve subjective well-being. Chapter 3 provides details on the PPIs to consider prescribing.

When individuals learn about the diversity of activities that are showing promise in positive psychology (PP) research, they might be overwhelmed. How should patients get started, especially if they have not had much experience with these types of activities? Psychology researchers recommend that individuals find "activity-fit," based on self-identified preferences (Layous et al 2015; Schuller 2011).

Medical practitioners might consider offering brief guidance to help narrow down the activities most likely to have a good activity-fit. The research to date provides lessons about the attributes of PPIs – "activity features," such as variety and dosing – which can affect results. Also, one needs to consider "person features," such as the individual's cultural background, prior experiences and personal needs.

Although we are still building the evidence base to guide best practices in the types of PPI prescriptions, supports, and resources that can produce improvements in emotional well-being, the research offers some tips to consider when recommending PPIs. Factors about the activity itself such as its variety, "dosage," and medium of delivery (e.g., in-person or online), and individual factors can influence the success of the intervention. The interplay between these factors determines the person-activity fit, according to a model developed by Layous and colleagues (2013). Individual factors include motivation, effort, self-efficacy, beliefs, baseline affective states, personality, social support, and culture. A number of these constructs should be familiar as part of health coaching (Chapter 6). Others are described below to help guide PPI recommendations.

In a busy practice, recommending an array of options (for example, by referring to the PERMA model) and allowing the individual patient to choose may be adequate. However, likelihood of intervention success could potentially be increased when a health team member works with the patient using the person-activity fit model to guide the selection process.

Guidance on Recommending Positive Psychology Interventions

When recommending PPIs, medical practitioners needs to consider a number of factors that can help increase the likelihood that the patient will successfully implement the PPIs, leading to improved positive emotions and emotional well-being. Among these factors are the variety of the PPIs planned, the patient's culture, the timing and "dosage" of the activities, the availability of social support to achieve and sustain the plan, and the patient's interest level and ease of doing the activities. The latter could potentially be boosted when the patient selects activities aligned with her signature strengths and personality.

Variety of Positive Psychology Interventions is Key to Sustaining Impact

Participating in a variety of positive activities is important to avoid hedonic adaptation–the observed tendency of positive emotions arising from a new positive experience to eventually revert to baseline emotions and mood. Activity changes lead to varied experiences and less adaptation (Sheldon 2006) and have the potential for longer term happiness effects. The rate of hedonic adaptation varies (Lucas et al 2003; Luhmann et al 2012; Lyubomirsky et al 2011) and might be slow for some individuals. Moreover, encouraging active appreciation and savoring of the positive emotion can slow adaptation (Lyubomirsky et al 2011; Sheldon & Lyubomirsky 2012). For example, thinking about what one appreciates about one's life partner/spouse can lead to satisfaction lasting long after the 2-year average adaptation period of married couples (Clark et al 2008; Lucas et al 2003).

Individuals should be encouraged to not only vary the activities, but also alter the focus of a particular activity. When doing gratitude practice, for example, an individual may change the focus to highlight various elements of their life, e.g., people, work, home, vacations, pets. Flow experiences (e.g., drawing, gardening, knitting) that are intentionally planned on a regular and frequent basis might need to be varied to maintain the level of reward and joy derived while doing them (Czikszentmihalyi 1990). Study participants who were asked to vary the acts of kindness that they did weekly reported greater increases in well-being than those who did the same kindness activity every week (Sheldon & Lyubomirsky 2012).

With emphasis on prescribing a variety of positive activities, Table 1 lists the common ones that can be easily implemented and alternated to vary the routine. A longer list of PPIs that can be prescribed is covered in Chapter 3 and summarized in Appendix B.

Table 1: Positive Activities

- Expressing gratitude–Writing letters of gratitude (Boehm et al 2011; Layous & Nelson et al 2013, Lyubomirsky et al 2011); thinking more gratefully; talking with a partner about good things that happened throughout the day; journaling three good things (Emmons & McCullough 2003)
- Feeling optimism–Thinking more positively about the future (Seligman 2006)
- Prosocial behavior–Doing acts of kindness or loving kindness meditation (Hofmann et al 2011)
- Forgiveness–Expressing forgiveness to those who have hurt us, writing letters of forgiveness to those who have passed away (Hendriks et al 2018)

Adapting Positive Psychology Interventions to Align with an Individual's Culture

When recommending PPIs, the individual's cultural background needs to be taken into account. Western cultures, namely the US, value individuals actively seeking out and planning activities that boost their happiness; some Eastern cultures do not support such active happiness pursuit (Boehm et al 2011). As with any recommended health behavior, the prudent practitioner should check with the patient in terms of the level of interest, support and readiness to undertake a change. Some patients might not be interested, others might even be offended, and still others who are open to new activities might not benefit due to the complex influence of cultural perspectives and expectations.

In one study, Asian-Americans randomly assigned to a positive activity did not achieve the same level of well-being increase as European-Americans who underwent the same random assignment (Boehm et al 2011). In cultures that operate by collectivist values, PPIs that involve acts of kindness and helping others might be more impactful on well-being than PPIs that target or emphasize personal well-being gain. A study of the effect of writing gratitude letters and performing acts of kindness in well-being showed that South Koreans fared better if they started with acts of kindness, whereas the reverse was true of the US participants. The researchers theorized that due to South Koreans' lower comfort in seeking support (Kim et al 2006), expressing gratitude for support might have led to feelings of guilt (Layous & Lee et al 2013).

Adjusting Timing and Dosage of Positive Psychology Interventions

Another factor influencing the level of benefit from PPIs is "dosing" (frequency and intensity of the activity). If someone performs an activity often, for extended amounts of time or not frequently enough, then the activity might not be effective. Gratitude practice and acts of kindness are types of PPIs that have been shown to be impacted by dosage. In one study, individuals who performed five acts of kindness all in one day derived greater increase in well-being than those who spread them out throughout the week (Lyubomirsky et al 2005). In another study, individuals who counted blessings once a week had larger gains in well-being than those who counted them three times a week (Lyubomirsky et al 2005). Hence, the timing and dosing of a PPI might be an essential factor to consider in order to develop a PPI plan that produces the greatest benefit. More research is needed to uncover special considerations for specific PPIs, such as the gratitude and acts of kindness examples.

Ensuring Social Support for the Positive Psychology Intervention

The likelihood of success to make a habit change increases with social support (Sullivan et al 2010). This factor also applies to individuals adopting positive activities. One study looked at the impact of social support when students were asked to write about their best selves. The group that was randomized to receive encouragement from peers about reaching their goals reported larger increases in positive affect than the group randomized to receive neutral information about resources available on campus (Layous et al 2013). Hence the practitioner needs to work with patients to identify social support to achieve PPI plans, in addition to the other benefits derived from social connection (as described in Chapter 2).

Aligning Positive Psychology Interventions with the Individual's Personality and Strengths

Research supports the common sense construct that people tend to spend more time on self-selected positive activities (Parks et al 2012). As with other health behaviors, people who have internal drive or interest in an activity might spend longer on the activity, do it more frequently and stick with it over time, thus deriving greater benefit (Parks et al 2012). With this knowledge and short of having best practices for the specific types of PPIs to recommend, busy practitioners can encourage patients to develop action plans based on personal interests. As noted above, some studies hint at the circumstances and conditions under which certain PPIs are more likely to produce improved outcomes (Lyubomirsky & Layous 2013). In the future, the field may evolve to allow for more specific prescriptions.

In the meantime, if patients ask for guidance, the practitioner can recommend selecting activities that align with an individual's personality and strengths. One approach is to use the individual's signature strengths (introduced in Chapter 6) to choose PPIs of greater interest and ease of participation or commitment.

Another approach is to use the individual's personality as a guide. An interesting question is whether different personalities correlate with different happiness levels. The Big Five personality traits and subjective well-being are cited as reciprocally influencing each other over time (Soto 2013). However, this framework might not be useful in selecting PPIs and developing positive activity plans.

How can medical practitioners help patients choose approaches to align with different personalities? One of the most widely used personality assessments is the Myers-Briggs Type Indicators (MBTI), which is based on an individual's preferred cognitive processes as described by the well-known psychologist Carl Jung (Lianov 2013). Of course, most busy medical practices will not have staff resources to implement this assessment and work directly with patients to personalize their plan. Hence, patients can be encouraged to do so on their own.

More research is needed to specifically guide positive activities according to these personality approaches. In the meantime, practitioners can suggest to interested patients that they consider using their personality preferences as one strategy for identifying potential good-fit PPI activities. Recognizing that the MBTI instrument has been criticized for its psychometrics (Pettinger 2005), it should not be used as a definitive assessment of personality, but rather as a starting point for developing self-knowledge that can be supplemented with reading the personality descriptions, reflecting on what aligns with their experiences, and further reading and exploration. The MBTI is lengthy, with 126 items, and is proprietary, often used by psychologists and career counselors. Shorter assessments can be found online, and a sample abbreviated tool is included in Appendix E.

Patients can explore their personality-based preferences, not only as an approach to identifying positive psychology-based activities for their healthy lifestyle action plans, but also as personal strengths. These preferences can be used like character strengths (Rashid 2015) to boost positive emotions and experiences, and support flourishing in a similar manner as used for harnessing Virtues in Action (VIA) signature strengths (Höfer et al 2019; Park & Peterson 2008) to achieve goals and a sense of well-being.

Intentional activities aligned with signature strengths and personal preferences can lead to a sense of competence and self-satisfaction, which can contribute to sustainability supported by perceived benefits of doing the activities (Deci & Ryan 2000; Sheldon et al 2001). Moreover, paying attention to individual personality-based preferences can help individuals arrange their activities in ways that promote positive emotions and steer away from situations that can lead to stress. For example, individuals who prefer planning and organizations can build routine PPIs into their lifestyles, avoiding the stress that could accompany a lack of structure. On the other hand, individuals who prefer spontaneity can allow themselves a variable and loose schedule to engage in PPIs, avoiding the stress of sticking with set activities at predetermined times. Another example is the influence of personality on one's preferences regarding frequency of social activities and the level of social interaction to avoid feelings of loneliness. Individuals who have extraversion preferences might need more social time to feel energized than those who have introverted preferences. Personality-based preferences can also be used to guide health behavior change and develop any healthy habit, including positive activities (Lianov 2013).

In acknowledging the need to customize PPIs, medical practitioners can encourage their patients to identify the "activity-fit" by exploring options based on culture, personality, personal strengths and other factors. These simple self-assessments are learning opportunities for patients to promote their well-being. Busy practitioners can point to resources, apps and supports for developing lifestyle changes most likely to be achieved and sustained. As machine learning and artificial intelligence evolve, a scientific approach to personalizing PPIs may be developed and become a standard patient-centric approach (Table 2) to assisting behavior change and lifestyle treatment plans.

Table 2: Factors to Guide the Selection of Positive Psychology Interventions

Intentionality of positive activities	Assist patients to choose positive activities that they can build into their lifestyles
Variety of positive activities	Ensuring a variety of positive activities for a patient's lifestyle can help decrease habituation
Dosing and timing of positive activities	Adjusting the timing and frequency of positive activities can help increase the benefit and potentially avoid resistance or negative effects. An example is ensuring that gratitude practice is not so frequent that resentment occurs. More insights about this aspect of positive activities will evolve as research progresses
Social support for positive activities	Encourage patients to identify a social contact who supports them in these positive activities
Cultural impact on the benefits of positive activities	Be sensitive to the patient's cultural background and preferences; avoid recommending positive activities that can backfire. Since this area of research is evolving, ask the patient about cultural preferences
Personality-based preferences for positive activities	Encourage patients to learn about their personalities by taking personality assessments or reading and self-observing preferences that can be leveraged to narrow down positive activities and identify achievable and sustainable ones

Additional Considerations

Some studies suggest that the impact on positive affect can be neutralized or even reversed when a person focuses too much on the results of activities undertaken to become happier. Framing PPIs as part of an overall healthy lifestyle with a goal of total well-being, without emphasis on happiness per se, might be a softer approach in making these recommendations.

Medical practitioners might wonder whether PPIs are feasible for all populations, including those from low socioeconomic demographics or disadvantaged backgrounds. Should PPIs be prescribed for patients when unmet social needs, other life priorities and/or low financial resources might be factors? The prudent approach, as with all medical prescriptions and recommendations, is to take into account each patient's unique situation, use clinical judgement about which healthy lifestyle elements are feasible, and check the patient's interest and readiness level to do them. As highlighted in Chapters 2 and 3, some PPIs are simple to do, do not take a lot of time and do not cost money (e.g., a few minutes in nature, gratitude practice). Simple PPIs have the potential to increase an individual's positive emotions, and, even if fleeting, these emotional states can help bolster the individual's capacity to build other resources. In fact, one might argue that disadvantaged populations are most in need of embracing simple interventions that increase positive emotions to offset stress, anxiety and depression they may experience, as well as to support flourishing.

Summary

Studies suggest that intentional activities can boost happiness and emotional well-being levels, despite genetic predispositions to baseline affect and life satisfaction levels. PPIs can be prescribed, and individuals can build positive activities into their lives as part of a healthy lifestyle. A variety of factors about these activities, as well as characteristics of the individual who is applying those activities, determine whether a good fit exists for the individual to fully engage in them and improve her emotional well-being.

In a busy medical practice, practitioners may direct interested patients to take self-assessment tools, read materials and access other resources that can help guide their positive activity selections. Some practices might have the staff capacity to designate a health team member/health coach to work with patients on personalizing positive activities and building emotional well-being action plans, in a similar way as, and along with, action plans for other health behaviors.

Resources

Myers Briggs Type Indicator: www.16personalities.com
Positive Psychology Center:https://ppc.sas.upenn.edu
Positive Psychology Program: www.positivepsychology.com
19 Best Positive Psychology Interventions and How to Apply Them: www.positivepsychology.com/positive-psychology-interventions
Virtues in Action Character Strengths: www.viacharacter.org

References

Bohem JK, Lyubomirsky S, Sheldon KM. A longitudinal experimental study comparing the effectiveness of happiness-enhancing strategies to Anglo-Americans and Asian-Americans. *Cognition Emotion* 2011;25:1263-1272.

Braungart JM, Plomin R, DeFres JC, et al. Genetic influence on tester-rated infant temperament as assessed by Bayley's Infant Behavior Record: Nonadaptive and adaptive siblings and twins. *Devl Psychol.* 1992;28:40-47.

Clark AE, Diener E, Georgellis Y, et al. Lags and leads in life satisfaction: A test of baseline hypothesis. *Economic J.* 2008;11:222-243.

Czikszentmihalyi M. *Flow: The Psychology of Optimal Experience*. New York, NY: Harper and Row, 1990.

Deci EL, Ryan RM. The "what" and "why" of goal pursuits: Human needs and the self-determination of behavior. *Psychol Inquiry* 2000 (4):227-268.

Emmons RA, McCullough ME. Counting blessings versus burdens: an experimental investigation of gratitude and subjective well-being in daily life. *J Pers Soc Psychol.* 2003;84(2):377–389.

Fredrickson BL, Cohn MA, Coffey KA, et al. Open hearts build lives: Positive emotions, induced through loving-kindness meditation, build consequential personal resources. *J Pers Soc Psychol.* 2008;92:1045-1062.

Heferon K. The role of embodiment in optimal functioning. In Joseph S. [Ed] *Positive Psychology in Practice, Promoting Human Flourishing, Education, and Everyday Life*, Hoboken, NJ: Wily, 2015.

Hendriks T, Schotanus-Dijkstra M, Hassankahn A, et al. The Efficacy of positive psychological interventions from non-western countries: A systemic review and meta-analysis. *Int J Well-Being* 2018;8(1).

Höfer S, Gander F, Höge T, et al. Special Issue: Character strengths, well-being, and health in educational and vocational settings. *Appl Res Qual Life* 2019. Doi.org/10.1007/s11842-018-9688-y

Hofmann SG, Grossman P, Hinton E. Loving-kindness and compassion meditation: potential for psychological interventions. *Clin Psychol Rev.* 2011;31(7):1126-32.

Kim HS, Sherman DK, Ko D, et al. Pursuit of comfort and pursuit of harmony: Culture, relationships and social support seeking. *Pers Soc Psychol B.* 2006;32:1595-1607.

Kok BE, Fredrickson BL. Upward spirals of the heart: Autonomic flexibility, as indexed by vagal tone, reciprocally and prospectively predicts positive emotions and social connectedness. *Biol Psychol.* 2010;85:432-436.

Layous K, Lee H, Choi I, Lyubomirsky S. Culture matters when designing a successful happiness-increasing activity: A comparison of the United States and South Korea. *J Cross Cultural Psychol.* 2013;44(8):1294-1303.

Layous K, Nelson SK, Lyubomirsky S. What is the optimal way to deliver a positive activity intervention? The case of writing about one's best possible selves. *J Happiness Stud.:* 2013;14(2):635-654.

Layous K, Sheldon KM, Lyubomirsky S. The prospects, practices, and prescriptions for the pursuit of happiness. In Joseph S. [Ed.] *Positive Psychology in Practice, Promoting Human Flourishing, Education, and Everyday Life* Hoboken, NJ: Wily, 2015.

Lianov L. *My Happy Avatar: Use Your Mobile Device and Personality to Transform Your Health.* Fair Oaks, CA: HealthType, 2013.

Lucas RE, Clark AE, Georgellis Y, et al. Reexamining adaptation and the set point model of happiness: Reactions to changes in marital status. *J Pers Soc Psychol.* 2003;84:527-539.

Luhman M, Hofman W, Eid M, et al. Subjective well-being and adaptation to life events: A meta-analysis. *J PersSoc Psychol.* 2012;102;:592-615.

Lykken D, Tellegen A. Happiness is a stochastic phenomenon. *Psychol Sci.* 1996;7:186-189.

Lyubomirsky S, Sheldon KM, Schkade D. Pursuing happiness: The architecture of sustainable change. *Rev Gen Psychol.* 2005;9:111-131.

Lyubomirsky S, Dickerhoff R, Boehm JK, et al. Becoming happier takes both will and a proper way: An experimental longitudinal intervention to boost well-being. *Emotion* 2011;11:391-402.

Lyubomirsky S, Layous K. Do simple positive activities increase well-being? *Curr Dir Psychol Sci.* 2013;22:57-62.

Park N, Peterson C. *Positive psychology and character strengths: Application to strengths-based school counseling.* Professional School Counseling 2018;12(2).

Parks A, Della Porta M, Pierce RS, et al Pursuing happiness in everyday life: The characteristics and behaviors of online happiness seekers. *Emotion* 2012;12(6):1222-1234.

Pettinger DJ, Cautionary comments regarding the Myers-Briggs Type Indicator. *Consult Psychol J: Pract Res.*2005;57(3):210-221.

Rashid T. Strength-Based Assessment. In Joseph S. [Ed.] *Positive Psychology in Practice, Promoting Human Flourishing, Education, and Everyday Life* Hoboken, NJ: Wily, 2015.

Roysamb E, Harris JR, Magnus P, et al. Subjective well-being sex specific effects of genetic and environmental factors. *Pers Indiv Differ.* 2002;32:211-233.

Schuller SM. To each his own well-being boosting intervention: Using preference to guide selection. *J Posit Psychol.* 2011;6:300-313.

Seligman MEP. *Learned Optimism, How to Change Your Mind and Your Life.* Vintage, 2006.

Sheldon KM, Elliot AJ, Kim Y, et al. What is satisfying about satisfying events? Testing 10 candidate psychological needs. *J Pers Soc Psychol.* 2001;80325-339.

Sheldon KM, Lyubomirsky S. Achieving sustainable increases in happiness: change your actions, not your circumstances. *J Happiness Stud.* 2006;7:55-86.

Sheldon KM, Lyubomirsky S. The challenge of staying happier: Testing Hedonic-Adaptation Prevention (HAP) model. *Pers Soc Psychol B*. 2012;38:670-680.

Sin NL, Lyubomirsky S. Enhancing well-being and alleviating depressive symptoms with positive psychology interventions: A practice-friendly meta-analysis. *J Clin Psychol*. 2009;65(5):467-487.

Soto C. Is happiness good for your personality? Concurrent and prospective relations of the Big Five with subjective well-being. *J Pers*. 2013;83(1). Doi: 10.1111/jopy.12081.

Sullivan KT, Pach LA, Bejanyan K, et al. Social support, social control and health behavior change in spouses. In Sullivan KT, Davila J. (Eds.). *Support Processes in Intimate Relationships*. New York City, NY: Oxford Press, 2010, p. 219-239.

Van Cappellen P, Rice EL, Catalino LI, et al. Positive affective processes underlie positive health behavior change. *Psychol Health* 2018;33:77-97.

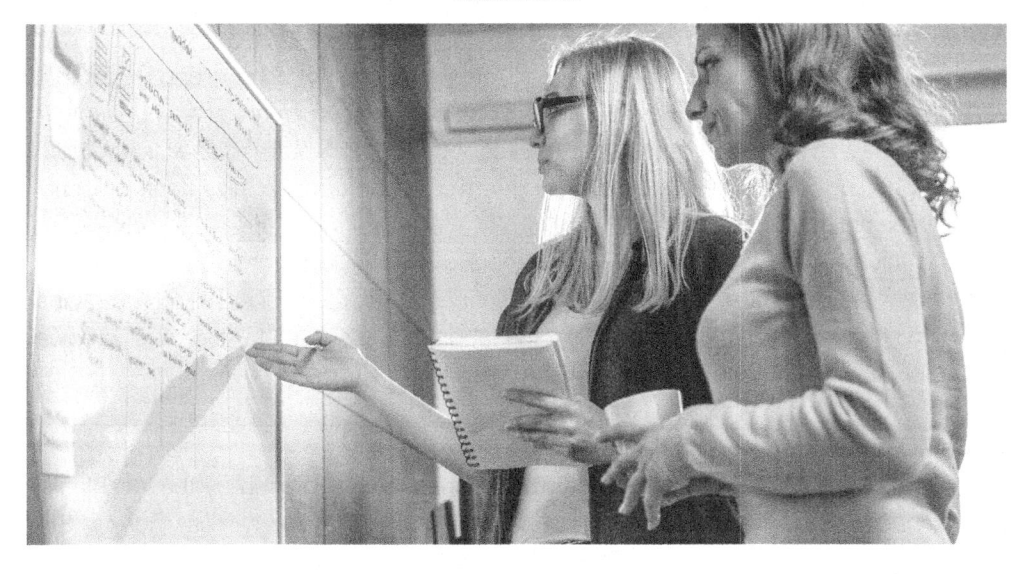

CHAPTER 8
Quality Improvement of Positive Psychology Strategies in Health Care
Liana Lianov

Chapter Goal 1 (Practical Application/Medical Case Example):
To apply positive psychology (PP) principles in a medical case example, including conducting patient assessments, developing health maintenance and treatment plans and facilitating healthy lifestyle action plans.

Chapter Highlights:
- PP principles, when fully implemented into health care practice, can permeate every aspect of care, including recruitment of new patients, conducting patient interactions, developing treatment plans, and ongoing follow-up of established patients.
- The medical practitioner (MP) can manage each patient through the lens of PP principles, with the support of the health care team, clinical processes, dashboards/health records, and digital technology.

Chapter Goal 2 (Continuous Quality Improvement):
To adapt continuous quality improvement (CQI) principles to measure and improve the integration of PP strategies into health care practice.

Chapter Highlights:
- CQI processes, including PDSA and rapid cycle improvement, root cause analysis, and process mapping, can be applied by health care practices to integrate PP principles and strategies into care.
- CQI can also be used to initiate, improve and sustain PP activities as part of health maintenance and treatment plans.

Medical Case Example

The orientation of a medical practice to emphasize lifestyle change and PP for total well-being can permeate every aspect of the practice from recruitment of new patients to ongoing follow-up with established patients. Previous chapters outlined specific methods for incorporating PP into practices, including formal and informal assessment, prescription of interventions, and follow-up.

In this chapter, we offer a case example of a lifestyle treatment approach that emphasizes positive activities. The details described in the case focus on the emotional well-being element of the visit. (Details of the laboratory assessment and other medical evaluation and interventions are not included here.)

Medical Case Example: Intake and Initial Encounter

Marlena H. is a 47-year-old Hispanic woman who was referred by the local family clinic for intensive lifestyle treatment of her diabetes and obesity (body mass index of 35). When she calls for an appointment, the front office staff explains that the clinic emphasizes healthy lifestyles and other well-being treatments. She is asked to complete a pre-visit total well-being assessment on a secure site online. Staff offers to mail her a paper copy if preferred.

The pre-visit assessment contains a medical history, medication list, family history, social history including prior trauma, review of systems, and current health habits. Lifestyle "vital signs" are checked, including nutrition and intake of fruits and vegetables; type, frequency and duration of physical activity; duration and quality of sleep; tobacco use; alcohol intake; and other substance use. She is asked to list her work history, types of regular social contacts, and hobbies and interests. The Patient Health Questionnaire-4 (PHQ 4) is included to screen for depression and anxiety, and a single-item stress screener asks her to rate her level of stress on a scale of 1 (least stressed) to 10 (most stressed). Her level of subjective well-being is assessed using the Satisfaction with Life Scale (SWLS).

On review of this assessment before the visit, we learn that Marlena H. takes metformin 500 mg and lovastatin 20 mg daily. She experiences headaches every other day and has occasional back pain, especially at the end of the work day. She does not list other medical conditions or history of trauma. She works as an office assistant for a tire company. She lives with her husband of 15 years and has a 12-year-old son. She lost her mother to diabetes complications three months ago and has been feeling down. Her PHQ-4 score is 5, stress level is 7, and her SWLS score is 15, perhaps indicating potential areas of concern, such as mild depression, moderate stress and below average satisfaction with life.

She walks about 30 minutes three times a week, mostly on the weekends. She eats wheat toast for breakfast, a salad for lunch, and fixes traditional Mexican meals for her husband and son for dinner, such as cheese enchiladas and chicken tacos. Her average vegetable and fruit consumption is about 3 servings per day. She gets about 6 hours of sleep per night. She does not smoke and on weekends she has a glass or two of wine. She does not have any regular hobbies, but enjoys knitting on her own, as well as with a knitting group once a month.

During her first visit, her BP is 150/90, pulse 68, and respiratory rate 18. The physician welcomes her into the practice and reinforces the message shared by the front office staff that the practice emphasizes a healthy lifestyle and total well-being. The physician asks whether she has any questions.

The physician then goes over the pre-visit assessment form with Marlena, obtaining additional information. Marlena admits to being stressed at work due to covering for another worker who recently quit and tensions with her husband about how to raise their son, who has been sneaking out to drink beer with school friends. She denies issues related to violence or abuse in the home. The physician also asks what she feels is going well in her life. Marlena reveals that despite current tensions with her husband, their relationship is strong; she also has many close relationships with extended family and friends who live nearby in her community, although she has not seen many of them as much as she would like, recently.

As described in Chapter 2, most lifestyle behaviors impact mental health and emotional well-being, including happiness. Hence, the results of a lifestyle and health behavior assessment can be viewed through the lens of physical and mental/emotional health. A correlation of adverse childhood events and other trauma with obesity and poor health habits calls for attention to these possible underlying factors. Although further research is needed on the impact of PPIs, including social support buffers, on health behaviors among patients with adverse childhood experiences and other trauma, the prudent medical practitioner may consider additional emphasis on PPIs to supplement the treatment plan, as well as promote positive emotions for total well-being (Felitti et al 1998; McEwan & Gregerson 2019). Table 1 summarizes the initial assessment.

Table 1: Initial Assessment: Items Related to Mental Health and Emotional Well-Being

Dashboard Item Related to Mental Health and Emotional Well-Being	Current Status	Assessment
BMI, waist circumference	BMI 35, waist 35	Obese – Obesity might be related to past trauma (e.g., early adverse childhood experiences, sexual abuse, domestic violence) and has potential to impact self-image, self-confidence and social relationships. Patient is a target for social interventions and PPIs (Felitti et al 1998; McEwen & Gregerson 2019)
PHQ-4	Score = 4; she denies suicidal ideation	Mild depression, anxiety (Kroenke & Spitzer 2009)
Stress level	7 on a scale of 1 to 10	Moderate stress at work and at home
Social contacts	Husband, son, knitting group	Not isolated, but has tensions currently with husband and son, and might have low positivity ratio in her life
Satisfaction with Life Scale	Score = 15	Below average life satisfaction (Pavot & Diener 2008)
Positive activities	Knitting, inconsistent activity on some weekends	Occasional "flow" experiences; no consistent positive activities
Sleep duration	6 hours	Inadequate sleep duration

Vegetable and fruit consumption, daily	Average 3 servings per day	Inadequate consumption for physical, mental and emotional health
Alcohol consumption	2 glasses wine/ week	Consuming above the recommended alcohol limit; and depressive symptoms can be exacerbated by alcohol (Ramsey et al 2005)
Tobacco use	Nonsmoker	Not smoking (as recommended for total well-being). Some data suggest smoking can exacerbate anxiety; also a complex interrelationship exists between smoking and depression (Mental Health Foundation, 2019)
Physical activity	30 min. walk 3 times a week	Inadequate physical activity level to counter her stress and mild depressive symptoms, and support weight and diabetes management

Medical Case Example Continued: Prescription and Agreed Upon Action Plan

The physician congratulates Marlena on her current habits of regular walking and eating fruits and vegetables and discusses next steps. The physician also describes the recommended lifestyle guidelines, and explains how improving lifestyle habits is the focus of her treatment plan, with the goal of getting her off the medications and enhancing her total well-being. The treatment prescription includes that she increase her vegetable consumption and walking, improve her sleep hygiene, and add some social and positive activities to her life.

Marlena and the physician identify her interest in increasing her vegetable consumption to 7 servings per day, increasing her walking to 30 minutes daily, attending her knitting group once a week, reaching out to meet with a girlfriend every other week, and starting the "three good things" exercise every week. The physician assesses Marlena's readiness to make changes, co-creating an action plan she is ready to do and assesses her confidence to implement the plan. She is confident at a level of 8 (on a scale of 1 to 10) that she will increase her walking to 5 times a week. She is also interested in starting the weekly "three good things" reflection exercise at a confidence level of 8. Her confidence level for adding a serving of vegetables to her dinners and to attend the knitting class weekly is 7. She also says she intends to reach out to her girlfriend to join the class. She admits that her interest and confidence in making changes to her sleep hygiene and alcohol consumption are low, at a confidence level of 4. Table 2 summarizes the prescription and the negotiated action plan.

Table 2: Prescription and Action Plan

Lifestyle Element	Prescription	Agreed Upon Action Plan
Social contacts	Increase positive social contacts, such as spending more time at the knitting group; manage communications with family to be constructive	Increase visits to knitting group weekly; reach out to a girlfriend weekly
Positive activities	Increase current positive activities to weekly; add new positive activity	Increase knitting to weekly; write down "three good things" weekly (Emmons & McCullough 2003)
Sleep duration	Increase sleep to at least 7 hours per night	Not ready to make a change
Vegetable and fruit consumption	Recommend whole food, plant-based diet	Add 1 or 2 servings of green beans or broccoli to dinner
Alcohol consumption	Eliminate alcohol consumption	Not ready to make this change
Physical activity	Increase walking to 30 minutes or more daily	Increase 30-minute walks to 4 times a week

Marlena develops an action plan for the changes she is confident at a level of 7 or higher she will achieve. Her current medication dosage will be adjusted after receipt of laboratory results. She is encouraged to monitor her weight and blood pressure and is referred to another health team member for coaching.

Busy practitioners and clinics can leverage the health team in the office or refer to external health coaches/other health professionals who offer coaching. Positive activities can be addressed using health coaching techniques in a similar manner as for other health behaviors. Examples are listed in Table 3. Chapter 6 describes positive psychology techniques for coaching.

Table 3: Sample Dialogue on Increasing Positive Activities

- "What activities do you do that improve your mood or make you feel good?"
- "How do you feel about adding or increasing positive activities in your life?"
- If the patient answers that she has an interest in adding or increasing these activities, provide information on how such activities can increase positive emotions, support health behavior change and have direct health benefits.
- If the patient affirms she will make these changes, inquire about the time frame: "When will you start making changes?"
- If the time frame is not near-term (next month or before next visit), provide resources and information, ask about a main barrier and encourage problem solving.
- If the time frame is near-term, ask whether she needs any assistance or needs specific resources.
- If the patient is ready to start immediately, negotiate an action plan, ask patient to write it down, check confidence level in achieving the plan, and note it in the medical chart for follow-up.
- If the patient says she is already doing positive activities, ask details, such as how often, for how long and with whom. Capture these activities in the medical record as positive health assets.
- If the patient is meeting a positive activity goal, encourage her to develop a relapse prevention plan for times when she gets busy or other life situations cause a lapse in the activity.

For most patients, a brief dialogue about elements of PERMA, regardless of level of readiness to make other changes, may be worthwhile, even in cases when an action plan is not developed. A medical practitioner may consider adding an asset list according to the PERMA framework, in addition to a problem list, in the medical chart notes. Such a list can serve as a reminder to discuss with the patient how these assets can help her achieve and sustain ongoing lifestyle interventions and treatment plans. As this type of PP approach grows in implementation, changes to electronic medical records could support quick data entry and dashboards that monitor these elements. The counseling time on positive activities can be billed by the physician or psychologist/behavioral coach as part of healthy lifestyle coaching to address medical conditions or incorporated in systems oriented toward value-based care.

Medical Case Example Continued: Follow Up

Follow up with Marlena focuses on all key health behaviors, including positive activities, with the goals of boosting the reinforcing link between these behaviors and emotional well-being (as described in Chapter 2), treating her diabetes, supporting weight loss, weaning her off medications, and enhancing her total well-being. Depending on Marlena's interests and personality (Chapter 7), she can be encouraged to try a variety of positive activities over time (Chapter 3), along with digital apps as appropriate (Chapter 12). Throughout the process, positive physician-patient interactions (Chapter 5) and PP strategies to facilitate health behavior change (Chapter 6) can support her in achieving these goals.

Quality Improvement Processes for Implementing Positive Psychology into Medical Practice

Altering current processes to integrate PPIs effectively into medical practice may seem daunting for busy physicians already experiencing the multiple, and at times conflicting, demands and realities of healthcare systems today. However, several frameworks for gradual modifications and enhancements to existing processes can be applied to ease the transition. The majority of these strategies draw principles and practices from the continuous quality improvement (CQI) methodologies.

CQI processes aim at effectively driving the best health outcomes (Jones 2015; Health Information Technology Research Center 2013). As a medical practice integrates intensive lifestyle treatments including PPIs, CQI can be conducted to evaluate the impact on the work flow of the health care team, the satisfaction of patients and the health team, and patient outcomes. Questions that can be answered using CQI processes should focus on practice changes that are planned or that have been made:
- What specific change are we trying to accomplish in our practice?
- How will we know that the change is an improvement?
- What adjustments to the initial change are needed to achieve the improvement? (AAFP; Coleman & Endsley 1999)

The health team can implement, evaluate and improve the key steps of changing a practice to embrace PP strategies (Chapter 4). The practice needs to evaluate whether newly adopted emotional well-being assessments are being completed by patients and whether the results are being used to prompt discussions on the topic and make PPI prescriptions. In the example of Marlena, the key CQI process focused on PPIs would evaluate the utility of information received from additional well-being assessment questions, as well as the adherence to and impact of increased social activities, and the "three good things" gratitude exercise. CQI can also look at how medical practice changes that incorporate PP affect the roles of health care team members and the overall satisfaction level of both patients and health team members. Also, the impact on clinical processes and flow would need to be evaluated.

Some medical practices might have the capacity to contribute to translational research by testing the impact of PP implementation on patient satisfaction, health behaviors and outcomes. Outcomes studies, however, often require large patient populations to enroll adequate numbers. Smaller practices can engage in studies that investigate the kind of clinical processes and flow needed to make prescribing and facilitating PPIs feasible for those settings. Research grants from foundations or research programs within health systems seeking to maximize health outcomes could support this work.

Even when conducting research projects is beyond the capacity of a health setting, interested practices can implement minor changes that incorporate PP strategies and test the impact on patient satisfaction, behavior change and outcomes as part of their overarching quality improvement goals. Common CQI methods can be applied to evaluate and facilitate the changes. For example, the Plan – Do – Study – Act (PDSA) cycle for designing, implementing, testing and revising clinical improvements can be used to evaluate small changes, such as the addition of a short happiness measure in routine intake assessments.

When a medical practice implements PP strategies during patient check-in, in the waiting room, in the examining room, or at checkout, some steps could be missed or slow the clinic flow. CQI processes can identify potential clinic flow issues and make adjustments. Root cause analysis, a method of identifying causal factors in a process or situation, and process mapping, an approach for understanding how components of a clinical process relate, are among the most common and useful CQI tools to analyze the problem (Agency for Health Care Research and Quality 2019). See Table 1 for examples of how CQI processes might be implemented.

In the case of Marlena, during her follow up visit, it is determined that she is not achieving her PPI action plan, because she has not identified someone to support her in achieving her goals. Process mapping discovers that the clinic does not have a staff person designated to follow-up on patients' action plans, including assessing and addressing social needs.

In a rapidly evolving healthcare environment, medical practices of the future can adapt digital technology and artificial intelligence to improve the quality of care (e.g., by automating process mapping); guide and support the redesign of practices; and personalize prescriptions. Currently, as for other health behavior change plans, technology can be helpful to track and support implementation of PPIs. Marlena, for example, could be asked to enter her "three good things" into an app or website (if she has easy access). Both she and her practitioner would have a record of how often she is doing this gratitude practice. With that data, they can investigate solutions to barriers. When are the time periods she is not doing her gratitude practice? Is there a pattern to those time periods?

CQI Culture Shift

The key to successfully shifting health care processes is to foster a culture that is open to, and supportive of, ongoing CQI with rapid cycle small changes, measurement and adjustments as needed. The health team needs to be flexible enough to embrace innovations and adjust roles and procedures based on the measurement results. A significant culture shift among some health teams may be required, as openness to failure during the innovation process is key to success (Shortell et al 1995). In addition, one or more staff need to take on the role of QI lead(s) to review the clinical processes and outcomes and obtain patient feedback. Involving patients in CQI is essential, because successfully promoting PPIs, as with other health-related behaviors, relies on patient-centric approaches (Shortell et al 1995).

Small medical practices might have more flexibility than large health systems for conducting ongoing tests of change to guide the redesign of work flow. On the other hand, they might be challenged by limited resources and staff to assist patients with developing and implementing PPI action plans. Even in the face of limited resources, the medical practitioner can orient the practice to embracing PP attitudes and strategies. The whole health team can use a patient-centric, positive interaction approach; and the practitioner can take brief moments during patient encounters to emphasize the need to address total well-being and add PPIs to lifestyle prescriptions. These changes, while seemingly small, can have powerful impacts on relationships with patients, health behaviors and practitioner satisfaction.

While modest changes that emphasize PP can be impactful, medical practices may require significant additional support to make major changes that address patients' well-being needs. Supportive reimbursement models, such as value-based care and systems focused on outcomes, may become early adopters of the PP-oriented approach to advance healthy lifestyle changes and improved health outcomes. Successful redesign may require maximally leveraging the available human, technological, material, and interpersonal resources to facilitate total well-being–including physical, social, mental, and emotional health (Locock 2003).

Summary

Table 4 offers some examples of how to adapt QI tools for assessing and implementing practice improvements in office clinical settings that aim to integrate PP strategies into care.

Table 4: CQI Processes Adapted for Integrating Positive Psychology Assessments and Interventions into Health Care

PDSA Cycle to Implement and Test a Change in Clinical Practice		PPI Integration Example
Plan	• Set an objective • Develop the plan (who, what, when, where) • Make predictions (hypothesis)	• Add 5-question Satisfaction with Life Scale (SWLS) to initial assessments • Office assistant (OA) will make this change to the online and paper assessment • Prediction: Most patients will complete assessment
Do	• Carry out the plan • Document • Begin to analyze the data	• OA makes the change
Study	• Complete data analysis • Compare to predictions • Summarize lessons learned	• After 4 weeks, QI staff analyze results and finds that only half of patients seen during this period completed questions
Act	• Ask what needs to be changed in the next cycle	• QI staff asks a sample of patients how to increase response. Response: Front office staff needs to encourage patients to complete assessment and explain that the total well-being goal is for all patients • Another option: conduct another PDSA using the 2-question SWLS
Rapid Cycle Improvement to Add a New Clinical Process		
What do we want to improve? What change should we test? What is the anticipated outcome?	• Quick planning • Small tests of change	Test of small change: • Health team member taking patients to team room asks them to list one positive activity in their lives; health team member notes answer in the record
Evaluate and determine the success rate Determine necessary changes to the new process	• Iterative process over several cycles • Planned time to look at each cycle and plan the next one	Evaluation • Patient responses are noted in chart, but physician is not making PPI recommendations • Brief interview with physician reveals she is not reading these notes during the clinical encounter New process: • PP-related questions are added to pre-visit assessment

Root Cause Analysis of a Break-Down in a Clinical Process or a Poor Outcome		
What is the underlying or predisposing cause of a problem in a clinical process?	• Ask four whys to understand what occurred upstream that led to the problem • Make an improvement change • Check results	Plan: • Add PPIs to routine lifestyle prescriptions; but QI staff finds only 65% of prescriptions include PPIs Analysis: • 1st why: Physician forgets new routine • 2nd why: Physician is not prompted to recommend PPIs • 3rd why: Standard prescription pad (online and paper) does not list emotional well-being component Improvement: • Add emotional well-being section on the standard prescription
Process Mapping of a Clinical Steps		
What steps in a clinical process led to a problem?	• Outline or draw the steps in a clinical process • Identify steps that led to a problem • Implement changes in the steps	Goal: • Each patient's health maintenance or lifestyle plan includes at least one PPI Problem: • QI staff note that only 45% of lifestyle plans include a PPI Analysis: • Process mapping shows that the health team member who completes (and reviews with patients) the action plans uses EMR notes from physician; EMR notes do not mention PPIs Solution: • Develop field in health maintenance section of EMR for PPIs

References

American Academy of Family Physicians: https://www.aafp.org/practice-management/improvement/basics.html

Agency for Health Care Research and Quality. US Department of Health and Human Services. Root Cause Analysis, 2019. https://psnet.ahrq.gov/primers/primer/10/root-cause-analysis; https://healthit.ahrq.gov/health-it-tools-and-resources/evaluation-resources/workflow-assessment-health-it-toolkit/all-workflow-tools/process-0

Coleman MT, Endsley S. Quality improvement: First steps. *Fam Pract Manag*. 1999;6(3):23-26.

Emmons RA, McCullough ME. Counting blessings versus burdens: an experimental investigation of gratitude and subjective well-being in daily life. *J Pers Soc Psychol*. 2003;84(2):377–389.

Felitti VJ, Anda RF, Nordenberg D, et al. Relationship of childhood abuse and household dysfunction to many of the leading causes of death in adults. The Adverse Childhood Experiences (ACE) Study. *Am J Pre Med*. 1998;14(4):245-58.

Fuemeler BF, Dedert E, McClermon FJ, et al. Adverse childhood events are associated with obesity and disordered eating: Results from a US population-based survey of young adults. *Trauma Stress*. 2009;22(4):329-333.

Health Information Technology Research Center. Continuous quality improvement (CQI) strategies to optimize your practice. The National Learning Consortium. April 30, 2013. Retrieved from: https://www.healthit.gov/sites/deafult/files/tools/nic_continuousqualityimprovementprimer.pdf

Jones K. Step by step: Proper planning essential for quality improvement. *Fresh Perspectives: New Docs in Practice*. AAFP. April 07, 2015. Retrieved from https://www.aafp.org/news/blogs/freshperspectives/entry/step_by_step_proper_planning.html, accessed April 2, 2019.

Kroenke K, Spitzer RL, Williams JB, et al. An ultra-brief screening scale for anxiety and depression: the PHQ-4. *Psychosom*. 2009;50(6):613-621.

Locock L. Healthcare redesign: meaning, origins and application. *Qual Saf Health Care*. 2003;12:53-58.

McEwen CA, Gregerson SF. A critical assessment of the adverse childhood experiences Study at 20 years. *Am J Prev Med*. 2019, Feb. 23. doi:10.1016/j.amepre.2018.10.16.

Moore M. *Coaching Psychology Manual*. Philadelphia, Pennsylvania: Lippincott Williams & Wilkins, 2015.

Mason PG, Butler CC. *Health Behavior Change, A Guide for Practitioners*. Edinburgh: Churchill Livingstone, 2010.

Mental Health Foundation. Smoking and mental health. Retrieved from https://smokefree.gov/challenges-when-quitting/mood/smokinh-depression and https://www.mentalhealth.org.uk/a-to-z/s/smokig-and-mental-health on April 2, 2019.

Pavot W, Diener E. The Satisfaction with Life Scale and the emerging construct of life satisfaction. *J Posit Psych*. 2008;3:137-152.

Ramsey SE, Engler PA, Stein MD. Alcohol use among depressed patients: The need for assessment and intervention. *Prof Psychol Res Pr*. 2005;36(2):203-207.

Shortell SM, O'Brien Jl, Carman JM, et al. Assessing the impact of continuous quality improvement/Total quality improvement: Concept versus implementation. *Health Serv Res*. 1995;30(2):377-01.

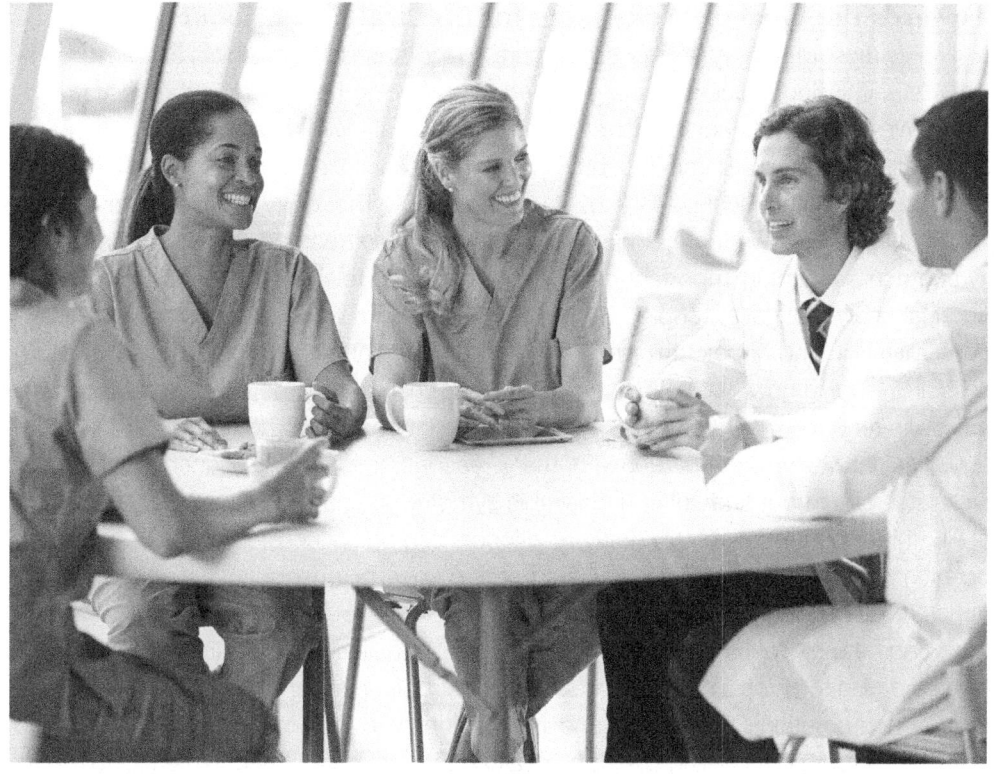

CHAPTER 9
Physician and Health Professional Well-Being Based in Positive Psychology
Kristen Collins

Chapter Goal:
To review how to implement positive psychology (PP) strategies and interventions that promote the well-being of physicians and health professionals (medical practitioners) in the face of the unique challenges of health care work.

Chapter Highlights:
- Lack of satisfaction, burnout and suicide among medical practitioners have increased in recent years.
- Strategies based on PP principles can be leveraged to boost and support medical practitioner well-being.
- Positive emotions, through positive interactions with patients and coworkers, and understanding and support of PP principles by senior leadership and the organizational culture not only improve satisfaction, productivity, and safety at work, but can foster positivity in other settings, with reinforcing effects.
- Medical practitioners can adapt the pillars of the PERMA model for their well-being.

Towards the Goal of Well-Being for Medical Practitioners

For most of society, and possibly more so for those in the medical and health professions, achieving success is the *goal* and experiencing happiness is the desired *outcome*. We work hard to achieve these results. We operate with a perpetual list of things to accomplish (i.e., land a dream job, buy an expensive car, lose ten pounds), thinking once we have successfully achieved them, we will be happy. The reality is quite the opposite.

Research shows that being positive and happy *first* actually drives our productivity and achievement in important areas of our lives (i.e., relationships, work, mental and physical health, longevity, coping with stress). Our brains work better when we're positive. Optimistic and hopeful thinking changes our perceptions and our ability to be successful, including how we manage hardships and challenges. People with these positive emotions tend to enjoy their jobs more and experience less burnout (Lyubomirsky et al 2005; Wright & Cropanzano 1998). For many reasons, medical practitioners tend to have high rates of burnout and suffer undesirable symptoms (Shanafelt et al 2012). Given this reality, it is important to identify how practitioners can be successful within an apparently counterproductive environment. Or, even better, how they might flourish in the face of apparently insurmountable odds.

Increasingly, patient treatment plans emphasize lifestyle medicine to prevent and reverse patients' chronic diseases. We can further define the landscape of lifestyle medicine by incorporating PP concepts and interventions into medical practitioners' lives and practices, including modeling the same health behaviors expected of patients. When we look at the convergence of lifestyle medicine and PP, it is profoundly evident that we live in a pivotal moment in time, providing us a unique opportunity to make exponential strides in creating health and well-being in our population.

Current State of Medical Practitioner Health and Well-Being

Medical practitioner burnout is widespread, common, and has damaging consequences. The grueling physical, mental, and emotional aspects of medical professions are integral and unavoidable aspects of the work. Deep systemic issues and limitations confound medical practitioners on a daily basis, and many times there is an unspoken resignation that things can't (or won't) change, and there is no use in trying to beat the system. Individuals who experience repetitive adverse situations may begin to feel the situations are unavoidable. Not uncommonly, these individuals develop the perception of having little to no control over their environment, and unconsciously become conditioned to feel defeated and helpless (Seligman 1972, 2011). Typical job and career demands can routinely place medical practitioners in this position, putting their health and well-being at risk. Expectations are high, and many times they can only be met if something else is sacrificed. Too often, the sacrifice is the physical and mental well-being of the practitioner.

Emotionally charged environments that often include sick or injured individuals rarely yield a healthy work-life balance. It takes effort to avoid burnout. Internal and external forces conspire against even those with the best intentions. However, physical, mental, and emotional energy are prerequisites to being engaged in a variety of contexts, (i.e., physically, emotionally, mentally, and spiritually) (Loehr & Shwartz 2003).

Burnout can be personally and professionally harmful for medical practitioners, and can have wide-ranging consequences. Physical and emotional exhaustion can be intense. Cynicism or sarcasm bristles, compassion for patients is lackluster, and the meaning or perceived value of caregiver work is jaded (Houkes et al 2011). Overall, burned out practitioners are less satisfied with their jobs, have lower well-being and life satisfaction, and they are more likely to be depressed, use drugs and alcohol, or die by suicide (Adikey et al 2018).

In this burnout-riddled environment, muddling through unscathed can seem impossible. The notion of *thriving* and *flourishing* personally and professionally could seem preposterous, or at the very least, quite daunting. However, it is possible. Incorporating wellness activities can be simple and short-term, more detailed and long-term, or anywhere in between. Moreover, focusing on well-being can be incorporated into busy lives.

Increasing Medical Practitioner Well-Being Benefits Patients

Patients can suffer, too. Medical practitioners are intimately and emotionally involved in patients' lives, including during times that may be confusing or scary for patients. In their own right, a patient can be taxing on the practitioner. They could have a complex injury or illness, or even a demanding personality. When medical practitioners are burned out, patients report receiving lower quality care and less satisfaction (Shanafelt et al 2017).

Consider a patient whose routine exam discovers something potentially serious. How would that patient feel if he or she was told there's a concern, it could be serious, and more tests need to be run? Definitely not happy or positive. Patients could feel more stressed, pessimistic, and helpless, which, unfortunately, can hinder healing (Seligman 2011). If the practitioner is tired, grumpy, just getting by with coffee and sugary junk foods, and has progressively become physically unhealthy, depressed, and disengaged, how might she behave during that patient interaction? Perhaps cold, abrupt, careless, or insensitive (Houkes et al 2011). Think about the impacts on the patient if the practitioner approaches the same interaction with a positive outlook, creative treatment plans, optimism about the results, and open-mindedness. The patient would likely take the frightening news better and leave feeling more confident in the practitioner and more hopeful in the recommended approach. (Fredrickson et al 2001; Seligman 2011).

Perceptions are important. Medical practitioners could be doing their patients a significant disservice if they are not functioning at their best. Additionally, prescribing aspects of a healthy lifestyle has a greater impact on the patient when the practitioner models the very behaviors and actions expected of patients (Adikey et al 2018; Lobelo & de Quevedo 2016).

Intentionally building positivity into daily life can help combat burnout. Positivity is transformational, builds capacity for growth, and establishes a healthy, flourishing life (Fredrickson 2009; Cameron et al 2003). Positivity helps medical practitioners be more open-minded and creative when diagnosing patients and finding solutions or creating action plans; negativity can restrict thinking and could lead to misdiagnoses.

A study mentioned in Chapter 5 and worth highlighting again is one that examined positivity and physician ability to review case information and diagnose patients. Merely "priming" the physician's positive emotions with candy (without consuming it) before analyzing the case information led to quicker and more accurate diagnostic and clinical insight into the case, as well as demonstrating less "anchoring" (being inflexible about patient diagnosis), even with conflicting information (Estrada et al 1997).

Positivity is contagious. Modeling positivity is important when interacting with patients; it's a tool that can help medical practitioners help their patients (as detailed in Chapter 5). When people demonstrate positivity through joy, gratitude, hope, or optimism, others feel it and begin to display it themselves (Fredrickson 1998).

To sum it up, if a practitioner walks into a patient's room with negativity, the patient is more likely to walk out with negativity. Instead, those who approach patient interactions with positivity can more easily improve their patients' lives.

Increasing Medical Practitioner Well-Being Benefits Medical Practices

Imagine a medical practitioner's typical workday and medical practice. What emotions are present? Is the work approached efficiently? Are the medical practitioner and team productive? Are the people there happy?

As burnout proliferates throughout a medical practice, the environment becomes toxic. Efficiency and productivity can drop. People can grow disengaged, and be absent or quit their jobs more often (Wright & Cropanzano 1998; Dyrbye et al 2019). Even more detrimental for everyone involved, these practitioners can make more medical and diagnostic errors, which could incur deleterious effects on patients and incur malpractice and litigation risks (Motluk 2018).

Well-being at work is important to take into consideration for both practitioners and medical practices. Not only does work influence a person's leisurely non-work activities (Sonnentag 2003), but life outside of work can influence a person's well-being and performance at work (Williams 1994), ultimately influencing business outcomes (Sonnentag 2003). Workplace strategies and interventions to address burnout can help organizations reduce the risks involved when the workforce is burned out (Panagioti 201; Shanafelt & Noseworthy 2017).

Feelings of little or no control in the workplace impact motivation, performance, and happiness (Snyder et al 2000; Sparr & Sonnentag 2008). Perceiving *some* control over the environment helps ease the stress and burnout associated with the job, which positively influences employees' well-being and life satisfaction (Thompson & Prottas 2006; Spector et al 2002).

Positive Organizational Scholarship

The field of positive organizational scholarship is the study of PP applied to the workplace (Cameron et al 2003). The large body of positive organizational scholarship research examines positive organizational outcomes, e.g., organizational efficiency, higher performing individuals and teams, better productivity, etc. (Cameron et al 2003; Losada 1999). These lessons are relevant to the health care workplace.

Organizational research is often derived from social and cognitive psychology premises, studying the "person" aspect within organizations. The organization-employee interaction is similar to an interpersonal social relationship (Eisenberger et al 1986) and employees tend to personify their organization (Levinson 1965). They form general beliefs about how much their organization cares about their well-being. This phenomenon is called perceived organizational support. Research on perceived organizational support shows that people (personified organization) help others (employees) who have helped them and the relationship becomes cyclical (Eisenberger et al 1986). When employees feel supported, they become more committed to their "relationship" with the organization and in return, help the organization achieve goals (Rhoades & Eisenberger 2002). Capitalizing on the social aspect of the organization-employee relationship to foster positive emotions can be valuable. Positivity in organizations can spread through interpersonal social interactions (e.g., between patients, coworkers, others in the building) as well.

The workplace can benefit from positive emotions (Cameron et al 2003). In working with patients, the same broaden-and-build and upward spiral effect as described in Chapter 2 can be seen in the workplace when co-workers co-experience positive emotions. In addition to fostering engagement and productivity in the workplace generally, positivity can dilute the negativity of a toxic workplace (Achor 2010; Fredrickson 2009; Snyder & Lopez 2003; Staw & Barsade 2006). Positive emotions are important *at work*, but it is also suggested that positive attitudes occurring in one context will contribute to positive emotions in other aspects of one's life, contributing to life satisfaction and well-being, which could be helpful for those focusing on work-life balance (Pinder 1998; Watson 2005).

Many improvements in organizational outcomes persist in the context of positive emotions and attitudes, such as job satisfaction and job involvement, as well as other desirable outcomes like goal attainment, effort, supervisor and coworker support, decision-making, coping responses, and personal resources (Bagozzi 2003; Fredrickson 2003; Fredrickson & Losada 2005; Pinder 1998; Watson 2005). Happy and healthy employees take fewer sick days, and they are actually *less* sick (Harter & Adkins 2015, Lyubomirsky et al 2005).

Resiliency, the ability to cope with a crisis and bounce back from it quickly, is a key component to intentionally foster in any workplace environment, particularly high-stress arenas such as healthcare. Barbara Fredrickson (2009) refers to resiliency as a "secret weapon". Given the challenging nature of the medical industry and profession, being resilient is extremely important. When resilient people are drained, psychological processes promoting personal assets serve to protect them from the negative impact of stressors, enabling them to recover better and faster (Fredrickson 2009; Stulbert & Magness 2017). Interestingly, groups and teams can also become collectively resilient and efficacious when they encounter problems or setbacks. Resilient organizations are more flexible and resourceful, and they learn from mistakes and make effective changes (Stulberg 2017).

Optimism is a strong predictor of work performance and facilitates employee problem solving by remolding problems as opportunities, resulting in employees that stay more engaged in challenges, set goals, and are better able to cope with stress (Cameron et al 2003; Snyder & Lopez 2003). Gratitude in organizations leads to positive outcomes like moral and prosocial behaviors in employees (Cameron et al 2003). As previously discussed, these positive emotions have a compounding positive effect on the workplace environment and employees (Fredrickson 2009).

Personal strengths are an important component of well-being (Seligman 2011). Leveraging personal strengths in the workplace can provide organizational benefits as well. We possess a human drive to build upon strengths and talents, which cultivates personal growth, task engagement, and organizational commitment (Colarelli et al 1987; Deci & Ryan 2001; Pinder 1998). Merely receiving feedback on one's personal strengths increases engagement, regardless of any developmental activities to build strengths (Asplund et al 2007; Buckingham & Clifton 2001; Rath 2007; Wagner & Harter 2007). When organizations or leaders invest in identifying and developing personal strengths for their employees, engagement is higher, productivity increases, employees feel more committed to the organization, and turnover decreases (Asplund 2007; Buckingham & Clifton 2001; Cameron et al 2003; Rath 2007; Wagner & Harter 2007). Medical practitioners who identify and harness their personal strengths on a daily basis and use them strategically long-term should also experience these same benefits.

Positive Psychology Interventions for Medical Practitioners

A movement toward a more healthful way of living for medical practitioners ultimately supports the field of lifestyle medicine and health care in general, as well as the goal of the field of PP–flourishing individuals and a resilient planet (Seligman 2011). Practitioners should develop the skills and grasp the opportunity to thrive in their professional and personal lives. When they invest in themselves and focus on increasing their well-being, the benefits are profound and far outweigh any challenges that may accrue in the effort to change.

Medical practitioners can apply the PERMA framework–positive emotions, engagement, relationships, meaning, and accomplishment (introduced in Chapters 3 and 6), for themselves, as well as their patients, to decrease the risk of burnout and increase the likelihood of flourishing (Seligman 2011).

Positive Emotions

One way to enhance well-being of both the medical practitioner *and* the patient is to do small things that increase positive emotions during patient visits. As detailed in Chapters 5 and 6, the patient experiences a host of benefits when the practitioner approaches the interaction positively and with compassion. The patient will understand the treatment better, adhere to treatment plans more, have less anxiety, and ultimately see improvement in their well-being (Martinez-Taboada et al 2017). Key to practitioner well-being is for individuals and teams working in healthcare organizations to engage intentionally in activities that enhance their workers' level of positive emotions. Consider the surgeon who plays upbeat music during surgery, the pediatrician who takes a moment to play with a young patient, or the healthcare team members who start their day together with a moment of reflection and gratitude. Momentary, meaningful positive interactions intentionally woven consistently and repeatedly into daily routines enhance job engagement and satisfaction and, ultimately, practitioner well-being.

Religion can be another useful tool to promote positive interactions and emotions. People who subscribe to religious beliefs or activities tend to have more positive affect and a greater sense of self-worth and coping skills, especially when contending with chronic illness or disability (Ellison 1993; Idler & Kasl 1997; Koenig et al 2012; Krause

2003). If religion is an important part of a patient's life, the practitioner could help generate these positive emotions by encouraging the patient to use their religion as a way to deal with challenges and stress. More details about positive patient-practitioner interactions are discussed in Chapter 5 and an expanded description of positive activities, including religious and spiritual activities that can improve well-being, can be found in Chapter 3.

Hope and optimism are important positive emotions, as well. An optimistic approach to life and work is a skill that can be cultivated (Lopez 2013; Seligman 2006). Active awareness of one's mindset and directing attention to indications of a positive future are essential for health providers, as with all individuals. Cultivating this skill set is essential in the face of experiencing the frustrations of health care organizational changes and witnessing colleagues or patients who are struggling.

Engagement

Research demonstrates that engagement or flow (introduced in Chapter 3) at work is positively related to health (Christian & Slaughter 2011). Engagement for medical practitioners may come from remaining mindfully present while conducting medical procedures or interacting with patients. However, for practitioners experiencing burnout, or those in highly restrictive environments, finding engagement at work might be challenging. Fostering work-life balance by finding engagement or flow in something outside of work, such as perfecting a craft or sport, might be more feasible. In an effort to benefit from social interactions, planning to do these activities with friends, family, or a social interest group could be reasonable in the context of busy lives. One could reap the benefits of engagement via work or life, or a combination of the two.

Relationships

Studies show that being or feeling isolated can have negative consequences. So much so that social isolation (actual and perceived) prompts pain centers in the brain similar to physical pain, and is a risk factor for mortality (Eisenberger 2012; Holt-Lunstad et al 2015). Strong social connections, having friends, and religion are associated with well-being and life satisfaction (Diener 1984; Idler & Kasl 1997; Krause 2003; Poloma 1990). Although medical practitioners interact with patients much of their work day, having friends *at work* can increase engagement, collaboration, and productivity, spur more positive interactions with patients and reduce turnover (Rath 2006). Additionally, busy practitioners who have religious and spiritual beliefs benefit from maintaining their participation in religious activities. Individuals engaged in such activities have been shown to have more social support and close relationships, and enjoy more socializing, leisure, and networking opportunities (Idler & Kasl199; Koenig et al 2012; Krause 2003).

In the context of busy healthcare teams, intentionally carving out opportunities for team members to connect and form strong relationships becomes key to ongoing engagement and, ultimately, performance of the team as a whole. The norms, cultures, and demands of different groups will vary, so it is important to consider the nature and types of activities that will promote the relationships and values important to the team's success. Whether teams decide to engage in regularly scheduled lunches for socialization, an annual offsite retreat to build team cohesion, after-hours social events, or some combination of these activities and more, critical to sustaining a team's well-being is to assess and plan how best to foster relationships and collaboration among team members.

Meaning

No matter the job, when people view their work as a calling, they tend to be more productive and successful. Meaningful work creates fulfillment and improves mental health, well-being, and longevity (Post 2005; Schwartz 2003, Wrzesniewski et al 1997, 2013).

When medical practitioners decided on medicine as a career, they may have wanted to help and heal people–a noble intention. However, given the education, training, and work demands required of practitioners, over time, motivation and meaning can wane. One strategy workers can use to reconnect with work-related meaning is to reflect on their "why" and rediscover their purpose through structured individual or team-based activities (Sinek et al 2017). For practitioners in particular, re-awakening compassion and identifying the role of compassion in their work can be a powerful tool that invokes and sustains meaning (Worline & Dutton 2017). Purposefully finding meaning in something *outside of work* or the medical profession is also a viable solution to combat burnout for practitioners and can also help contribute to work-life balance (Cameron 2003; Post 2005). Volunteering in the community is a way many people find fulfillment, perhaps even in a role that could benefit from medical knowledge or experience. Practitioners with school-age children can consider becoming involved in school activities or sports to balance family needs and instill a sense of meaning.

Religious worldviews can also provide a powerful source of meaning. Religious perspective can help people frame negative or tragic events, malicious people, and even the existential meaning of life, in the context of a higher purpose, or the will of God. Individuals who draw on their religion during personal or health crises cope better, are more optimistic about their recovery, and can reframe these experiences as chances to find meaning and spiritual growth (Ellison 1993; Idler & Kasl 1997; Koenig et al 2012; Krause 2003; Paloma & Pendleton 1990; Seligman 1990).

Accomplishment

Individuals possess a need to be strong and competent, and they strive to achieve that need. This self-determined behavior explains a person's need to seek challenging situations or experiences that offer opportunity to achieve mastery and meet goals (Deci & Ryan 1985). Feelings of accomplishment or achievement mean using skills and effort to realize success (Seligman 2011). The healthcare arena provides many opportunities to strive for mastery and goal attainment. This goal achievement may take the form of expanding one's learning through new certifications (such as becoming certified in lifestyle medicine!) or other educational achievements; enhancing one's expertise beyond medical knowledge to acquire acumen in business-related competencies, soft skills, or leadership development; becoming involved and taking leadership roles in professional organizations; or developing the experience and expertise to achieve promotions or other professional advancements.

Alternatively, medical practitioners may be unable to move personal goals forward given the environment or nature of the work, or they may have already achieved mastery in their professional role. For those who have accomplished their major life goals, looking for sources of accomplishment outside of work may offer greater well-being boosts. Seeking work-life balance by mastering an instrument or a challenging musical score, entering local competitions, learning a new physical skill, or writing a blog may bring feelings of accomplishment.

Positive and Other Activities That Improve Well-being

Positive activities can have short- and long-term positive effects on well-being and happiness (Parks & Biswas-Diener 2013; Sin & Lyubomirsky 2009; Smit et al 2013). Practicing the core healthy lifestyle modifications, including positive activities, is key to boosting medical practitioners' well-being and can enable the modeling of positive health behaviors for patients.

One does not need to incorporate all recommended activities into life to improve well-being. Each adopted positive activity conveniently provides exponential benefits, thanks to the broaden-and-build effect (Fredrickson et al 2001). Specific to lifestyle modifications, a meta-analysis found that there are *incremental reductions* in all-cause mortality with each additional lifestyle behavior someone incorporates into their life. Table 1 outlines a process for gradually incorporating strategies to enhance well-being and Table 2 in the next section includes information about the positive impacts of medical practitioner well-being.

Table 1: Positive Psychology and Healthy Lifestyle Interventions for Medical Practitioner Well-Being

Gain the knowledge	Identify activities	Put it to practice
• Review the positive psychology interventions (PPIs) and healthy lifestyle approaches in Chapters 2 and 3 and in this chapter, including the PERMA framework. • Consult the positive psychology tools and resources in Chapter 12 and in the appendices. • Envision how to leverage interventions personally or with friends, family, coworkers.	• Start by choosing 2-3 activities to focus on for personal well-being.	• "Test" some of the interventions to implement with patients, as well as for personal well-being. • Choose 1-2 activities to implement in the workplace with peers, staff, teams, etc. • Add more or alternate activities as comfort-level increases.

Summary

Due to the multitude of impacts, high levels of medical practitioner burnout and suicide are gaining greater attention. As healthcare organizations and systems are beginning to make changes that support medical practitioners, practitioners can advocate for the kind of changes they'd like to see (Chapter 10). At the same time, practitioners can increase their life satisfaction by implementing positive activities, e.g., those in the PERMA framework and other activities (Chapter 3) and healthy lifestyle approaches (Chapter 2) discussed in this handbook. These approaches are feasible, even for busy practitioners. Many of the PP approaches do not take extra time, but require a shift in mindset to notice the good in one's life and look for joy in simple interactions with co-workers, family, and friends. Small changes can have far-reaching benefits for practitioners, their families, their patients, and the healthcare/medical practices.

Table 2: Medical Practitioner Well-Being and Its Impacts

Studies of medical practitioner burnout have uncovered many major stressors:
<ul><li>Electronic health records</li><li>Quality patient care vs. time restraints</li><li>Demands of third-party payers</li><li>Various laws, procedures, policies</li></ul> <ul><li>Workload</li><li>Documentation requirements</li><li>Patient time constraints</li><li>Potential malpractice litigation</li></ul>

Practitioner burnout can be detrimental to their health, patients, and medical practices:

Provider	*Patient*	*Practice*
• Low quality of life • Little to no work-life balance • Personal relationship problems • Emotional exhaustion • Substance abuse • Depression and anxiety • Suicide or suicide ideation	• Receives low quality care • Low patient satisfaction with care • Perceives that the provider lacks empathy • Lack of patient-physician collaboration on treatment plans	• Medical or diagnostic errors • High turnover • Risks of litigation

Benefits happy people experience include:

- Mental and physical health
- Life satisfaction
- Well-being
- Broad thinking
- Flexibility
- Creativity
- Finding new ideas, and possibilities
- Optimism
- Resiliency
- Better decision-making
- Open mindedness
- Better social behaviors
- Increased work performance

When medical practitioners focus on their personal well-being compared with those who have low levels of well-being, positive impacts on patients can result in:

- Helps patients cope better, handle stress, and recover faster and better
- Higher well-being related outcomes before, during, and after illness, surgeries, and medical crises
- Lower levels of stress hormones
- Higher levels of opioids and dopamine
- Lower blood pressure
- Better immune functioning
- Less cardiovascular disease and infectious illness
- Better cancer outcomes
- Better coping tactics for patients with post-traumatic stress disorder
- Increased longevity

(Achor 2010; Dyrbye et al 2019; Fredrickson 2003; Fredrickson 2009; Fredrickson 2010; Friedberg et al 2013; Lyubomirsky et al 2005; Seligman 2006; Seligman 2011; Shanafelt 2009; Shanafelt & Noseworthy 2017; Shananfelt et al 2017)

References

Achor S. *The Happiness Advantage: The Seven Principles of Positive Psychology That Fuel Success and Performance at Work.* New York: Crown Business, 2010.

Adikey A, Bachu R, Malik M, et al. Factors related to physician burnout and Its consequences: A review. *Behav Sci (Basel).* 2018;8(11):98.

Ashby F, Isen A, Turken A. A neuropsychological theory of positive affect and Its influence on cognition. *Psychol Rev.*1999;106(3):529-550.

Asplund J, Lopez SJ, Hodges T, et al. *The Clifton StrengthsFinder® 2.0 Technical Report: Development and Validation.* The Gallup Organization, Princeton, NJ; 2017.

Bagozzi RP. Positive and negative emotions in organizations. In: Cameron KS, Dutton JE & Quinn RE, eds. *Positive Organizational Scholarship*. New York: Oxford University Press, 2003:176-193.

Bodai BI, Nakata TE, Wong WT, et al. Lifestyle medicine: A brief review of its dramatic limpact on health and survival. *Perm J.* 2017;22:17-25.

Buckingham M, Clifton DO. *Now, Discover Your Strengths*. New York: Free Press, 2001.

Cameron KS, Dutton JE, Quinn RE. eds. *Positive Organizational Scholarship: Foundations of a New Discipline*. New York: Oxford University Press, 2003.

Christian M, Slaughter J. Work engagement: A meta-analytic review and directions for research in an emerging area. *Acad Manag Proc.* 2011;2007(1):1-6.

Cohen J, Jenkins DJA, Talpers S, et al. A low-fat vegan diet improves glycemic control and cardiovascular risk factors in a randomized clinical trial in individuals with type 2 diabetes. *Diabetes Care* 2006;29(8):1777-1783.

Colbert AE, Mount MK, Harter JK, et al. Interactive effects of personality and perceptions of the work situation on workplace deviance. *J App Psychol.* 2004;89(4);599-609.

Colarelli SM, Dean R, Konstans C. Comparative effects of personal and situational influences on job outcomes of new professionals. *J App Psychol.* 1987;72(4), 558-566.

Deci EL, Ryan RM. *Intrinsic Motivation and Self-Determination in Human Behavior*. New York: Plenum Press, 1985.

Diener E. Subjective Well-Being. *Psychol Bull*. 1984;95(3);542-575.

Dyrbye LN, Johnson PO, Johnson LM, et al. Efficacy of the Well-Being Index to identify distress and stratify well-being in nurse practitioners and physician assistants. *J Am Assoc Nurse Pract*. 2019:1.

Eisenberger N. The neural bases of social pain: Evidence for shared representations with physical pain. *Psychosom Med*. 2012:74(2):126-135.

Eisenberger R, Huntington R, Hutchison S, et al. Perceived organizational support. *J App Psychol*.1986;71(3);500-507.

Ellison G. Religious involvement and self-perception among black Americans. *Social Forces*. 1993;71(June):1027-1055.

Estrada CA, Isen AM, Young MJ. Positive affect facilitates integration of information and decreases anchoring in reasoning among physicians. *Org Behav Hum Dec*. 1997;72(1):117-135.

Fredrickson BL. What good are positive emotions? *Rev Gen Psychol*. 1998;2(3):300-319.

Fredrickson BL. The role of positive emotions in positive psychology. *Am Psychol Assoc*. 2001;56(3):218-226.

Fredrickson BL. Positive emotions and upward spirals in organizations. In: Cameron KS, Dutton JE, Quinn RE eds. *Positive Organizational Scholarship*. New York: Oxford University Press; 2003:163-175.

Fredrickson B, *Positivity: Top-Notch Research Reveals the Upward Spiral That Will Change Your Life*. New York: Three Rivers Press, 2009.

Fredrickson BL, Mancuso RA, Branigan C, et al. The undoing effect of positive emotions. *Motiv Emot*. 2000;24(4):237-258.

Fredrickson BL, Tugade MM, Waugh CE, et al. What good are positive emotions in crisis? *J Pers Soc Psychol*. 2001;84(2):365-376.

Fredrickson BL, Losada MF. Positive affect ad the complex dynamics of human flourishing. *Am Psychol*. 2005;60(7):678-698.

Friedberg MW, Chen PG, Van Busum KR, et al. *Factors Affecting Physician Professional Satisfaction and Their Implications for Patient Care, Health Systems, and Health Policy*. RAND Corporation, 2013.

Harter J, Adkins A. *Engaged Employees Less Likely to Have Health Problems*. 2015:1-6. http://www.gallup.com/poll/187865/engaged?employees?less?likely?health?problems.aspx?version=prin.

Holt-Lunstad J, Smith TB, Baker M, et al. Loneliness and social isolation as risk factors for mortality: a meta-analytic review. *Perspect Psychol Sci*. 2015 Mar:10(2):227-37.

Houkes I, Winants Y, Twellaar M, et al. Development of burnout over time and the causal order of the three dimensions of burnout among male and female GPs. A three-wave panel study. *BMC Public Health* 2011;11(1):240.

Idler EL, Kasl SV. Religion among disabled and nondisabled persons: cross-sectional patterns in health practices, social activities, and well-being. *J Gerontol: Soc Sci*. 1997:52B(6):S294-305.

Koenig HG, King DE, Carson VB. *Handbook of Religion and Health*. New York: Oxford University Press, Inc., 2012.

Krause N. Religious meaning and subjective well-being in late life. *J Gerontol: Soc Sci*. 2003:58B(3):S160-170.

Levinson, H. Reciprocation: The relationship between man and organization. *Adm Sci Quart*. 1965;9(4).

Lobelo F, de Quevedo IG. The evidence in support of physicians and health care providers as physical activity role models. *Am J Lifestyle Med*. 2016;10(1):36-52.

Loehr J, Schwartz T. *The Power of Full Engagement: Managing Energy, Not Time, Is the Key to High*

Performance and Personal Renewal. New York: The Free Press, 2003.

Lopez SJ. *Making Hope Happen: Create the Future You Want for Yourself and Others*. New York: Atria Books, 2013.

Losada M. The complex dynamics of high performance teams. *Math Comput Model*. 1999;30(9-10):179-192.

Lyubomirsky S, King L, Diener E. The benefits of frequent positive affect: Does happiness lead to success? *Psychol Bull*. 2005;131(6):803-855.

Martinez-Taboada, C, Hermosilla, D, Delgado L, et al. Improving communication between physicians and their patients through mindfulness and compassion-based strategies: a narrative review. *J Clin Med*. 2017;6(3):33.

Motluk A. Do doctors experiencing burnout make more errors? *Can Med Assn. Journal* 2018;190(40):E1216-E1217.

Parks A, Biswas-Diener R. Positive interventions: Past, present and future. In: Kashdan T, Ciarroch, J [Eds.] *Bridging Acceptance and Commitment Therapy and Positive Psychology: A Practitioner's Guide to a Unifying Framework*, 2013:140-165.

Pinder CC. *Work and motivation in organizational behavior*. Upper Saddle River, NJ: Prentice Hall, 1998.

Poloma MM, Pendleton BF. Religious domains and general well-being. *Soc Indic Res*. 1990;22:255-276.

Post S. Altruism, happiness, and health: it's good to be good. *Int J Behav Med*. 2005;12(2):66-77.

Rath T. *The People You Can't Afford to Live Without: Vital Friends*. New York: Gallup Press, 2006.

Rath T. *Strengths Finder 2.0*. New York: Gallup Press, 2007.

Rhoades L, Eisenberger R. Perceived organizational support: A review of the literature. *J App Psychol*. 2002;87(4):698-714.

Schneider MF. Driving continuous improvement in plant safety. *Occup Hazards* 2007;36-40.

Schwartz M, Carroll A. Corporate social responsibility: A three-domain *approach*. *Business Ethics*. 2003;13:503-530.

Seligman M. Learned helplessness. *Annu Rev Med*. 1972;23:407-12

Seligman MEP. *Learned Optimism: How to Change Your Mind and Your Life*. New York City, NY: Vintage, 2006.

Seligman M. *Flourish: A Visionary New Understanding of Happiness and Well-being*. New York, Free Press, 2011.

Shanafelt TD. Enhancing meaning in work: A prescription for preventing physician burnout and promoting patient-centered care. *J Am Med Assoc*. 2009;302(12):1338-1340.

Shanafelt TD, Boone S, Tan L, et al. Burnout and satisfaction with work-life balance among us physicians relative to the general us population. *Arc. Intern Med*. 2012;172(18):1377-1385.

Shanafelt TD, Noseworthy JH. Executive leadership and physician well-being: Nine organizational strategies to promote engagement and reduce burnout. *Mayo Clin Proc*. 2017;92(1):129-146.

Shanafelt T, Goh J, Sinsky C. The business case for investing in physician well-being. *JAMA Intern Med*. 2017;177(12):1826-1832.

Sin N, Lyubomirsky, S. Enhancing well-being and alleviating depressive symptoms with positive psychology interventions: A practice-friendly meta-analysis. *J Clin Psychol*. 2009;65(5):467-487.

Sinek S, Mead D, Docker P. *Find Your Why: A practical guide for discovering purpose for you and your team*. New York: Penguin, 2017.

Smit F, Bohlmeijer E, Bolier L, et al Positive psychology interventions: a meta-analysis of randomized controlled studies. *BMC Public Health*. 2013;13(1):1.

Snyder CR, Lopez SJ. (Eds.). *Positive Psychology: The scientific and practical explorations of human strengths.* Thousand Oaks, CA: Sage Publications, Inc., 2007.

Sonnentag S. Recovery, work engagement and proactive behavior: A new love at the interface between non-work and work. *J App Psychol.* 2003;88(3):518-528.

Sparr JL, Sonnentag S. Feedback environment and well-being at work: The mediating role of personal control and feelings of helplessness. *Eur J Work Organ Psychol.* 2008;17(3):388-412.

Spector P, Cooper C, Sanchez, J, et al. Locus of control and well-being at work: how generalizable are western findings? *Acad Manag J.* 2002;45(2), 453-466.

Staw BM, Barsade SG. Affect and Managerial Performance: A Test of the Sadder-but-Wiser vs. Happier-and-Smarter Hypotheses. *Adm Sci Q.* 2006;38(2):304.

Stulbert, B, Magness, S. *Peak Performance: Elevate Your Game, Avoid Burnout, and Thrive with the New Science of Success.* New York: Rodale Books, 2017.

Tawfik DS, Profit J, Morgenthaler TI, et al. Physician burnout, well-being, and work unit safety grades in relationship to reported medical errors. *Mayo Clinic Proceedings.* Nov 2018;93(11):1571-1580.

Thompson CA, Prottas DJ. Relationships among organizational family support, job autonomy, perceived control, and employee well-being. *J Occup Health Psychol.* 2006;11(1):100-118.

Wagner R, Harter JK. *12: The Elements of Great Managing.* New York: Gallup Press, 2006.

Wallace JE, Lemaire J. On physician well-being: You'll get by with a little help from your friends. *Soc Sci Med.* 2007;64(12):2565-77.

Watson D. Positive affectivity: the disposition to experience pleasurable emotional states. In: Snyder CR, Lopez SJ. (Eds.). *The Handbook of Positive Psychology.* New York: Oxford University Press; 2005:63-73.

Williams KJ, Alliger GM. Role stressors, mood spillover, and perceptions of work-family conflict in employed parents. *Acad Manag J.* 2018;37(4):839-868.

Worline M, Dutton JE. *Awakening Compassion at Work: The Quiet Power That Elevates People and Organizations.* Oakland, CA: Berrett-Koehler Publishers, Inc., 2017.

Wright TA, Cropanzano R. Emotional exhaustion as a predictor of job performance and voluntary turnover. *J Appl Psychol.* 1998;83(3):486-493.

Wrzesniewski A, McCauley C, Rozin, P, et al. Jobs, careers, and callings: people's relations to their work. *J Res Pers.* 1997;31:21-33.

Wrzesniewski A, Lobuglio N, Dutton JE, Berg JM. *Job Crafting and Cultivating Positive Meaning and Identity in Work.* Vol 1. Emerald Group Publishing Limited, 2013.

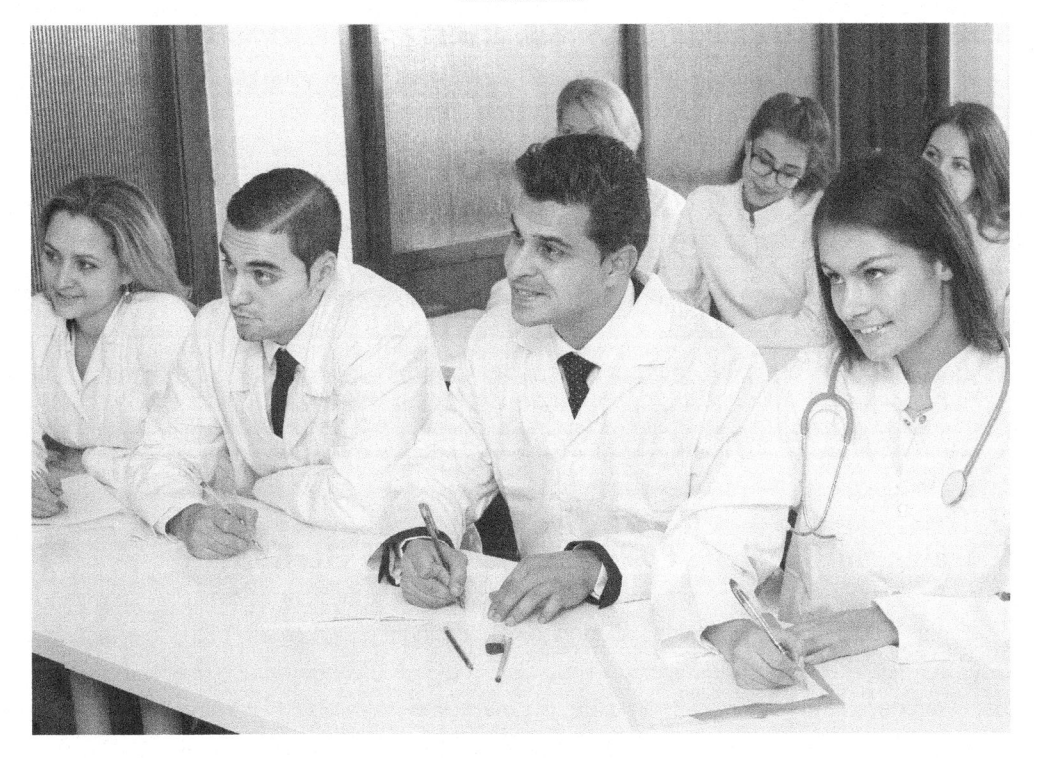

CHAPTER 10
Positive Psychology in Medical Education and Beyond: Teaching, Modeling, Integrating and Advocating
Grace Caroline Barron

Chapter Goal 1 (Teaching):
To teach and model positive psychology (PP) approaches and principles for health care team members, residents, and students throughout professional education/training.

Chapter Highlights:
- Focusing on self-awareness optimizes use of PP techniques in the PERMA framework during clinical care.
- Connecting with personal meaning early during medical and health professional training programs boosts the well-being of learners and their capacity to apply PP principles.
- Integrating PERMA principles into narrative questions during clinical encounters need not take more time, yet can shift the depth of understanding of patient needs and advance patient-centered care.
- Harnessing character strengths is essential to becoming an effective health professional, as well as enhancing personal well-being.
- Embracing PP does not mean ignoring the spectrum of emotions experienced by learners, professionals and patients, but rather fully acknowledging them (emo-diversity) and addressing them with a positive approach.

Chapter Goal 2 (Advocacy):
To assist physicians and health professionals to advocate for resources for, and attention toward, emotional well-being in their health care settings, such as in value-based health care models.

Chapter Highlights:
- Creating safe and open environments and using effective communication strategies can help advocates/champions open dialogues about the critical role of PP in patient care.
- Early adopters and advocates of PP can advocate for its integration into health care through open discussions, personal application, role modeling, and inspiring/engaging colleagues and patients to explore its benefits for well-being and effective health care.

Learning and Teaching Positive Psychology in Health Care

"It is not about what you have to offer but what the other can receive." A seasoned professors' wisdom speaks to the importance of honoring the individuality of the learner (Vigilante 2019). PP helps individuals flourish by clarifying their unique characteristics and using that awareness to build a more optimal life. Knowing who you are, how you work, where you are in your life and what matters to you maximizes learning. This approach cultivates vitality, motivation, a growth mindset and grit or the wisdom to know when to cut loss and change course. Awareness of limitations and leanings optimizes learning and the ability to thrive.

The PERMA (positive emotion, engagement, relationships, meaning, and accomplishment) template for optimal living (Chapters 3, 6, and 9) takes unique forms for each person. By applying personal insight to PERMA, students are able to take control of their development and ultimately apply what they learn to their patients (Duckworth et al 2005).

Personal and Professional Development Pathways through Positive Psychology

Teaching the basic tenets of PP to professional learners builds resilient caregivers and whole-person care practitioners. Medical literature is replete with articles about the need for humanism, interpersonal medicine, relationship-centered care. Robust physicians and other health professionals are poised for professionalism and operate out of their best selves (Lown 2016).

Intentional focus on emotional well-being can be learned, and the associated behaviors are both life-long skills and inner resources. PP practices can help one cope with systemic dysfunction, private loss, disaster management (Schulenberg 2016) and other stressors. Finding meaning, one of the PERMA components, is a way of managing under taxing circumstances (Park 2016). Teaching trainees to maximize meaning–by connecting with a personal calling, for example–and emphasizing other PP tenets early on is useful for well-being.

For each learner, knowing and owning which subjects and mentors bring positive emotion, deep engagement, excitement and meaning is helpful. Goals can change as one develops, but self-awareness helps with selection and adaptation. Faculty at Dell

Medical School use interactive, small group teaching, discussion, exercises and self-directed learning to facilitate the integration of new concepts and help students choose their professional paths. Students are asked to explore personal character strengths and leanings and to reach out to faculty for enrichment and support. Role-modeling is considered one of the best ways to enhance natural character strengths and chart a meaningful path (Branch et al 2014). Well-chosen mentors can make a large difference.

Alignment between natural self and professional choice has the potential to foster satisfaction, flow and competence. However, sometimes we don't know who we are or how we work. Unknowingly, we might select a situation or follow the lead of an influential person that leads us into challenges that neither move us nor fit our nature. The self-awareness and self-possession associated with PP practices create honed identity and capacity as well as greater joy and personal empowerment. Operating out of our strengths is an effective way to stay engaged and motivated to refine our skills as life-long learners and resilient caregivers (Goodman et al 2017). We might be surprised, stretched and strengthened if we focus on "lesser strengths" sometimes, too.

Teaching Techniques That Emphasize Positive Psychology

Opportunities for strength-based interventions naturally arise in the clinical encounter if one has the PP template in mind. Introducing students to this clinical perspective early on can deepen their understanding of the technique. Integrating PERMA with the traditional diagnostic questions need not take extra time. Instead, the emphasis shifts to awareness or receptivity and picking up on a spontaneous utterance that reveals who the patient is and what they care about. The approach involves a narrative rather than a formulaic inquiry. For example, a formulaic question might be about duration of symptoms. The narrative question might be, "Oh, you seem to light up when you talk about fishing with your son. Is this something you really love to do?" Engagement, positive emotion, relationships, meaning, and perhaps hope and accomplishment are addressed in this inquiry (Vigilante 2019).

Asking patients about what is important to them, who is there for them and for whom they deeply care, lets the health care team know about social supports and sources of pleasure. This dialogue gives people the opportunity to talk about losses, loneliness, desires, values and interests. These variables matter for self-care and treatment recommendations. Dell Medical School students are taught that addressing these apparently small details in a person's story can make a large difference in health care. Does someone with a broken shoulder have to walk an energetic dog? Is there a friend or family member who can change a bandage? Is there a beloved pastime (e.g., knitting, biking, watching movies) that can absorb the patient's mind or provide distraction, even for just a little while?

Students see that when we ask people what they love to do, what deeply engages them, initial surprise and then eagerness to answer is a common reaction. Drawing, cooking, gardening, walking with a friend or working with a certain colleague can highlight a day. A question about what makes someone feel lighthearted often brings a smile. A common answer to, "What makes you laugh?" is, "My dog!" Play, or non-goal directed pleasurable activity, is connected to positive emotion, the first of the PERMA principles.

Positive emotion is connected to learning and motivation, better self-care and clinical satisfaction (Fredrickson 2005). Students see that seeming banter about "soft stuff" in the clinical encounter is really a facilitator of rapport, adherence, meaning and elevated moments, all of which serve care. By using humanity and spontaneity in our approach to those we care for, good things happen. Even if the news is dire, feeling cared for can make patients believe that they have received good treatment (Beach 2006).

Teaching trainees to inquire about where people are in their lives outside their illness enhances meaning and well-being for both parties. What brings positive emotion, engagement, relationships, meaning, accomplishment, hope and allows for a better day? Clinicians enjoy the meaningful moments that arise from questions of this sort, because listening, hearing and even being awed by another person's story is a pro-social behavior. Pro-social behaviors elevate mood and do not need to take extra time. They can be incorporated into the exam. One may be amazed by a tale of resilience, a fascinating history, a talent, skill or interest not documented in the chart that speaks volumes about who someone is and what moves them.

The curiosity, respect and emotional connection in the clinical encounter stimulated by this level of awareness benefits both parties. Pro-social behavior in the clinical encounter can be an antidote to stress, and useful for hardworking caregivers (Chancellor et al 2018). Burnout is less likely if a greater frequency of meaningful moments, created by meaningful interactions with patients, characterizes the day. If one is awed, feels engaged, connects to others, and feels effective, it makes for a better day and a more satisfying practice. Teaching trainees these techniques early on so they see with their own eyes how adding depth to the encounter works for both caregivers and care-seekers is a way to change culture and bring positive psychology into healthcare.

Asking someone about their character strengths and passions brings the vitalized part of the self into the room. It can push the reset button in the psyche. Can-do attitudes or growth mindsets, adherence and self-care skills emerge (Dweck & Yeager 2019). Medical trainees are likely to be drawn to humanistic positive psychology conversations. We are a self-selected group of compassionate people who like to care for others effectively. Compassion is commonly defined as a sympathetic consciousness of another's distress *with the desire to alleviate it.*

Perhaps we had a trying event early on, or perhaps we possess an inborn love of humanity that inspired us to take action. Either way, being effective includes integrating our natural character with our situation and helping those we care for do the same. The social determinants of health play a significant role in well-being, and intra-psychic, extra-psychic and situational factors intersect in complex ways. Knowing about how an individual works and the context in which they function, helping them own and cultivate their inner strengths is good medicine. The PERMA template and principles, integrated into the clinical encounter, enhance care and inspire learners and patients alike. Many students see this information as meaningful and are enlivened by learning and discussing it.

Character Strengths in Medicine and in the Classroom
Character

Character has become a much talked about topic as can both serve patients and protect practitioners (Leffel et al 2018). But what does it mean, how does it work and how can we teach it? After exploring the scientific, spiritual, psychological and philosophical literatures, Peterson and Seligman identified 24 character strengths or qualities (listed in Chapter 6) that allow for "the good life" (Park 2009). Chapters 6 and 7 noted how these character strengths can be used to support health behavior change coaching and select PPIs.

How can we use the VIA survey to teach character to trainees? Trainees can access the survey, print out results and bring them to class. In a small group classroom setting, the students might share their results as well as a meaningful, personal story of how they used their strengths. At Dell Medical School, such sharing sometimes leads to tears and sometimes laughter, but students are always moved by the experiences of others. This activity elicits deep listening skills, compassion, empathy and stronger bonds. The experience shows how whole-person narratives and knowing someone more deeply facilitates greater understanding, communication and connection. The medium is the message. PERMA comes to life–the embodiment of the principles, the lived manifestation of the theory–in the classroom. This exercise allows students to explore PERMA personally and see how it can have an impact on resilience (Seligman 2011).

An important point is that positive emotion does not always involve ebullience or happiness. Insight, truth, feeling safe, self-expression and knowing someone cares conjure a positive feeling. The positive emotion may be more about acceptance and contentment than euphoria; decreased anxiety and a sense of calm, as opposed to high energy and vitality moments; or it can involve the freedom to share a secret in a journal (Berry & Pennebaker 1993) or to a person. Also, for trainees, learning how to read affect and feelings and respond appropriately is important. They need not fear emotion and should be encouraged to embrace emo-diversity. Tears can have a positive component if they stem from a feeling of trust, and can help an individual's psyche evolve. Working through something in the company of others brings with it a certain kind of hope. Just touching a hand, standing with, or looking deeply into the eye of someone who has to bear difficult news or adjust to a new diagnosis can help, even if there is uncertainty and no concrete action that can be taken. Students tend to be interested in these ideas and how they apply to clinical work.

Stating the policy "What is said in here, stays in here" sets the frame for trust among students and mentors and seeds a connected, caring group. Students tend to be rapt when they listen to their peers share a story of early loss of a parent, living without means, managing an impairment, or witnessing tragedy. They gain an awareness of the role of positive emotion, engagement, relationships, meaning and accomplishment, whether in the form of triumph over difficulty or achievement of excellence.

In teaching character, you can work from a strengths-based, as opposed to a deficit-based, model (Gander et al &2016). Teaching involves facilitating existing strengths through modeling and other means (Branch et al 2014). Each student has greater and lesser character strengths and virtues. The goal is to own one's character strengths and know they can expand with intention, circumstances, and development and via influential role models. The recipe for flourishing that includes leveraging strengths includes insight, selection skill, some control over one's environment, self-mastery (Duckworth & Seligman 2017) and well-chosen mentors.

In the Classroom

Interactive exercises, minimal slide content, and a teacher who can be him or herself in front of a group of people and has experiential knowledge of the subject foster learning. Sensitivity to cultural diversity helps create a psychologically safe learning space. Encouragement to explore mistakes openly (with critique rather than judgement) seeds growth and a deeper grasp of how to manage complexities. Critical thought processes, decorum, high expectations, integration rather than regurgitation of material, and skill in responding to emotions, affects and feelings in those we care for are classroom fare (Doukas et al 2010).

Context Matters

Natural style dictates, but contexts and psychological conditions influence, learning. Receptivity improves when worries abate. Being able to concentrate on the work rather than having to manage others' impressions of you is useful. Evaluations are a reality, but an evaluative process that allows for dedication to the skill over the grade enhances learning. Pass/fail instead of letter grades, for example, has been shown to increase emotional well-being in medical students (Dyrbye et al 2019). Medical students are often younger and in possession of precious, healthy ideals that energize them. Residents may benefit from an emphasis on supportive cultures and strong relationships. Faculty and staff can be strengthened by a focus on meaning, purpose and calling.

True Practice

Finally, PP mindsets and behaviors involve practice. Once one is enlightened to PERMA, the next step is to make chosen practices habitual. So, when we give "tips" (as listed at the end of this chapter), it is with the caveat that they require intention and practice. When it becomes a habit, it takes root in the inner life and can be a resource to draw upon in times of stress for learners, caregivers and care-seekers.

The true practice of teaching can, perhaps, be summed up in the acronym TEACH:

T: Trust the natural abilities of the learner and bring them forth.
E: Encourage openness about questions and errors.
A: Allow yourself to reveal your own puzzlements. Model love of inquiry.
C: Create opportunities to integrate positive psychology questions into clinical conversations.
H: Hear what students have to say.

A few exercises to promote emotional well-being of learners are suggested in Table 1.

Table 1: Ten Emotional Well-being Exercises for Learners

1. Journal about three good things that happened today and your role in them just before sleep.

2. Conjure gratitude on a regular basis. Think less about mortality, more about positive energy.

3. Create brief, warm, friendly interactions with peers or colleagues a few times per day.

4. Fashion a gratitude site in your workplace or school. Establish a place where people can post comments and observations about the good work of colleagues.

5. Explore and honor your character strengths and your PERMA (viacharacter.org)

6. Foster a growth mindset. Cultivate grit, but know when to quit, if it is not a good fit.

7. Volunteer. Altruism lifts moods and meaningful projects make people happy.

8. Maintain loving relationships, even if it means keeping in touch with texts.

9. Connect to your sense of meaning, purpose, awe, and transcendence.

10. Reckon with, accept, manage and sublimate the negative effects of intensive use of your character strengths–the shadow-side of yourself (viacharacter.org).

Advocating for Inclusion of Positive Psychology in Health Care
The Elephant in the Room

While the idea of emotional well-being is a non-controversial topic, the implementation of these practices into everyday healthcare is another matter. We face resistance. Time crunches, crises, medical emergencies, psychological urgencies, the emphasis on evidence-based medicine, a suspicion of the "soft stuff," and longstanding personal and systemic habits create a reluctance to shift ways and means. This resistance is understandable. Respect of a person's resistance and recognizing many of its causes is an empathic act and can create receptivity. We can enter the dialogue and seek to understand their psychological position. People often dislike what they do not understand. Focus on concrete things, like tests and formulas, can be easier than the somewhat amorphous vagaries of emotional exchange or personal values. Yet, clinical conversations that elucidate values, positive emotion and meaning to the patient carry measurable weight.

How can we convince leaders, learners and medical education stakeholders to integrate PP (Slavin et al 2012) and to embrace the challenge of adding one more thing to do or think about in the clinical encounter? This situation is especially challenging if that addition feels soft, unnecessary or abstract. Stories, conversations and human connections that touch the emotions can be an effective way to raise awareness. Difficult dialogues, crucial conversations and truthful talk can deepen that integration, and data/scientific evidence helps (Seligman 2005).

When we encounter individuals who resist the view of health care that emphasizes healthy lifestyles, PP and well-being to address patients with a whole system approach, we can meet them where they are. What are leaders and stakeholders worried about? What are they after? What are their misgivings? "Understand before you argue," a wise colleague once said. That can easily be morphed to "Understand before you advocate." Where can this discussion take place? Online? Town halls? Workshops? Gatherings in the workplace? Many options exist. Create a safe and open environment, use effective communication strategies and employ significant empathy. Offer nurture, viscerally and psychologically.

Terminology and the Shadow Side

Sometimes people bristle at the term positive psychology, because it seems to fly in the face of the seriousness of matters that emerge in medical care. The term seems, on its surface, to dismiss the "negative" (Held 2002). People might feel PP is somehow not addressing or honoring the "shadow" side of things–the challenges, difficulties and hardships we all face at times. When recommending PPIs, it is important for medical practitioners to convey that inclusion of this approach does not dismiss deeper concerns and that pain, struggle and despair must be addressed. After grappling with negatives, the positives can follow. And sometimes, when patients are open to a reverse approach, PPIs can prompt the upward spiral of positive emotion and garner resources to help address the negative.

The poet Robert Frost wrote that, "The best way out is always through" (Untermeyer 2002). PP approaches help patients. This perspective should directly address the skepticisms and concerns of educational stakeholders.

Transcendency and Awe Helps in Living and Learning

Medical practitioners advocating on behalf of the importance of PP can remind learners that this field is the scientific study of human flourishing, or the strengths and virtues that enable individuals, communities and organizations to thrive. Instead of focusing on experiential deficits, it mobilizes personal assets to identify ways of coping with (not dismissing or denying) challenges, and identifying life-affirming activities. It allows for moments of transcendence, awe and the sublime (Lewis 2018).

Above all, the practice of PP is the practice of uplifting humanity, a celebration of the strengths and virtues of individuals that allow triumph and transcendence in everyday life. PP is a branch of the humanities that has an important place in medical education. Re-grounding medicine in its historic humanity is appropriate for training learners and inspiring practitioners. PP arose out of the thinking of the great humanistic psychologists Abraham Maslow (Peterson & Park 2010), Rollo May (1967), Carl Rogers (Kramer 1995), and Viktor Frankl (1962), thinkers, researchers and clinicians who prioritized human welfare and potential. This knowledge helps learners identify with such ideals, values and methods.

An acronym to highlight the actions that incorporate PP into advocacy leadership is ADVOCATE:

Key Points for Advocating

A: Assure stakeholders that the soft stuff has impact.
D: Divulge data on efficacy.
V: Voice unspoken skepticism that stakeholders may have.
O: Open up an interactive dialogue.
C: Create ways for people to observe positive psychology in action.
A: Allow for resistance and introduce new alternatives with patience.
T: Thank people.
E: Engage, create positive emotion, form relationships, conjure meaning and accomplish!

Such advocacy leadership is essential to propel the integration of relevant aspects of PP into lifestyle medicine and health care in general.

Summary

Highlighting positive psychology in teaching, modeling and advocacy can facilitate the achievement of these goals, as well as leverage PP for promoting total well-being in health care.

Resources

Positive Psychology in Medical Education Course Outline (Syllabus in the appendix)

Values in Action Survey: http://www.viacharacter.org/Survey/Account/Register

References

Beach MC, Inui T. Relationship-centered care. A constructive reframing. *J Gen Inter Med.* 2006;21 Suppl 1:S3-8.

Berry DS, Pennebaker JW. Nonverbal and verbal emotional expression and health. *Psychother Psychosom.* 1993;59(1):11-19.

Branch WT, Jr., Chou CL, Farber NJ, et al. Faculty development to enhance humanistic teaching and role modeling: a collaborative study at eight institutions. *J Gen Intern Med.* 2014;29(9):1250-1255.

Chancellor J, Margolis S, Jacobs BK, et al. Everyday prosociality in the workplace: The reinforcing benefits of giving, getting, and glimpsing. *Emotion (Washington, DC)* 2018;18(4):507-517.

Doukas DJ, McCullough LB, Wear S. Reforming medical education in ethics and humanities by finding common ground with Abraham Flexner. *Acad Med.* 2010;85(2):318-323.

Duckworth AL, Steen TA, Seligman ME. Positive psychology in clinical practice. *Ann Rev Clin Psychol.* 2005;1:629-651.

Duckworth AL, Seligman MEP. The science and practice of self-control. *Perspect Psychol Sci.* 2017;12(5):715-718.

Dweck CS, Yeager DS. Mindsets: A view from two eras. *Perspect Psychol Sci.*.2019: 1745691618804166.

Dyrbye LN, Sciolla AF, Dekhtyar M, et al. Medical school strategies to address student well-being: a national survey. *Acad Med*. 2019. doi:10.1097/ACM.0000000002611

Frankel V. *Man's Search for Meaning*. Boston, Massachusetts: Beacon Press, 1962.

Fredrickson BL, Losada MF. Positive affect and the complex dynamics of human flourishing. *Am Psychol*. 2005;60(7):678-686.

Gander F, Proyer RT, Ruch W. Positive psychology interventions addressing pleasure, engagement, meaning, positive relationships, and accomplishment increase well-being and ameliorate depressive symptoms: a randomized, placebo-controlled online study. *Front Psychol*. 2016;7:686.

Goodman FR, Disabato DJ, Kashdan TB, el al. Personality strengths as resilience: A one-year multiwave study. *J Pers*. 2017;85(3):423-434.

Held BS. The tyranny of the positive attitude in America: observation and speculation. *J Clin Psychol*. 2002;58(9):965-991.

Kramer R. The birth of client-centered-therapy: Carl Rogers, Otto Rank, and the beyond. *J Humanist Psychol*. 1995;35(4):54-110.

Leffel GM, Oakes Mueller RA, Ham SA, et al. Project on the good physician: further evidence for the validity of a moral intuitionist model of virtuous caring. *Teach Learn Med*. 2018;30(3):303-316.

Lewis B. A medical sublime. *J Med Humanit*. 2018, Sep 6. doi:10.1007/s10912-018-9536-y.

Lown BA. A social neuroscience-informed model for teaching and practising compassion in health care. *Med Educ*. 2016;50(3):332-342.

May R. *Love and Will*. New York City, NY: WW Norton & Company, 1969.

Park CL. Meaning making in the context of disasters. *J Clin Psychol*. 2016;72(12):1234-1246.

Park N, Peterson C. Character strengths: Research and practice. *J Coll Character* 2009;10(4).

Peterson C, Park N. What happened to self-actualization? Commentary on Kenrick et al. *Perspect Psychol Sci*. 2010;5(3):320-322.

Seligman ME. Building resilience. *Harvard Bus Rev*. 2011;89(4):100-106, 138.

Untermeyer L, Frost R. *Robert Frost's Poems*. New York City, NY: St. Martin Press, 2002.

Schulenberg SE. Disaster mental health and positive psychology: Considering the context of natural and technological disasters: An introduction to the special issue. *J Clin Psychology* 2016;72(12):1223-1233.

Seligman ME, Steen TA, Park N, et al. Positive psychology progress: empirical validation of interventions. *Am Psychol*. 2005;60(5):410-421.

Slavin SJ, Schindler D, Chibnall JT, et al. PERMA: a model for institutional leadership and culture change. *Acad Med*. 2012;87(11):1481.

Vigilante FW, Personal Communication, 2019.

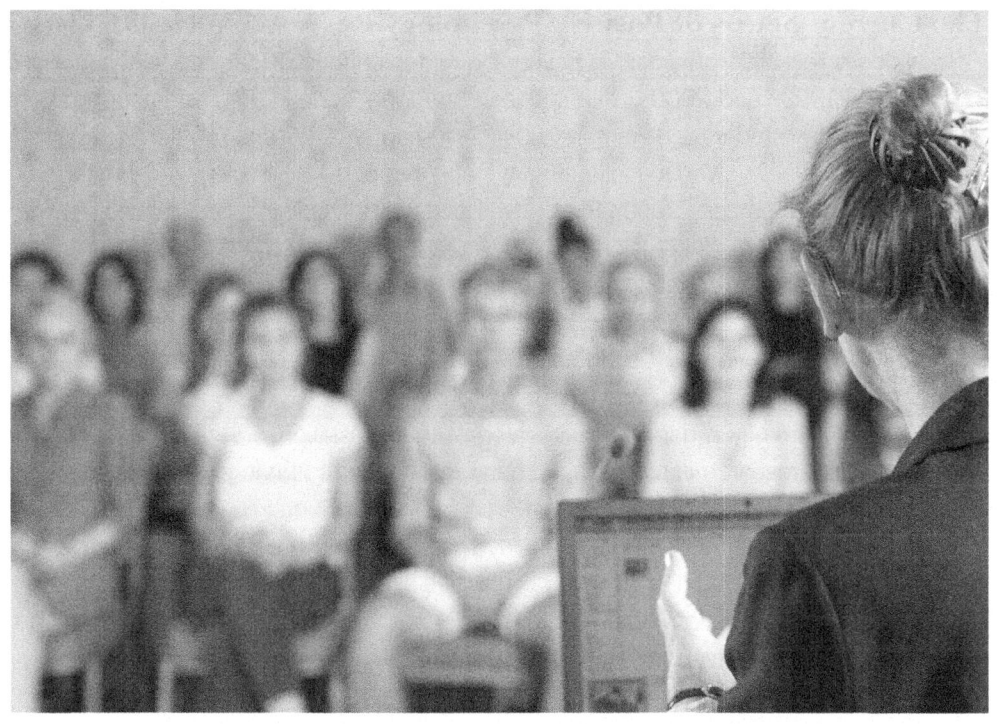

CHAPTER 11
Positive Psychology Research in Health Care Settings
Rachel Millstein and Liana Lianov

Chapter Goals:
- To describe status of positive psychology (PP) research in care care settings, including current research gaps for interventions that promote health outcomes
- To recommend roles for medical practitioners (MPs) in advancing PP research for health care settings

Chapter Highlights:
- Translational research in health care settings is needed to test PP principles and activities shown to be useful in other settings.
- MPs can partner with research societies and local universities to advise research teams on hypotheses and research methods relevant to health care settings.
- MPs and PP researchers and clinicians should consider attending cross-discipline research conferences.
- MPs can refer to published meta-analyses to see the current scope of the PP research in various clinical populations.
- MPs can collect PP measures to test feasibility and results of positive psychology interventions (PPIs) that are recommended as part of healthcare.
- While the evidence-base is strengthened, MPs can consider applying research-informed PP practices to support health goals.

The Current Status of Positive Psychology Research in Health Care

Modern research on positive psychology interventions (PPIs) began to gain attention in the 1990s and 2000s, with studies commonly done in the general population or healthy college students (Seligman 2004; Seligman et al 2005). The field of positive psychology (PP) has evolved to include many patient populations in clinical trials (Bolier et al 2013; Sin & Lyubomirsky 2009). PPIs have been tested in clinical populations ranging from mental health (e.g., depression, anxiety disorders, post-traumatic stress disorder) to multiple cancers (e.g., breast, ovarian, colorectal) to chronic diseases (e.g., type 2 diabetes, cardiovascular disease) (Chakhssi et al 2018). PPIs are also being developed to help promote healthy behaviors for use in primary care settings with patients in a pre-disease state, such as metabolic syndrome (Millstein et al 2017).

There is currently a gap in the research at the translational level, which is largely because the PPI research is still forming. Early trials show that it is possible to improve positive psychology constructs and positive emotions through simple activities. The intervention research has encompassed many types of positive psychology "exercises," which rely on simple thought or behavioral activities aimed at promoting constructs such as happiness, life satisfaction, optimism, gratitude, positive affect, perseverance, joy, and meaning making (Sin & Lyubomirsky 2009).

Three recent PPI meta-analyses have found encouraging (small to moderate) effect sizes in favor of using these interventions to improve well-being and reduce depressive symptoms (Bolier et al 2013; Chakhssi et al 2018; Sin & Lyubomirsky 2009). Thus, while intervention research is in its early stages, the initial findings are promising in the domains of well-being and depression. Current research is exploring the use of PPIs to promote health behaviors (e.g., physical activity, healthy diet, medication adherence) among patients with cardiovascular disease, type 2 diabetes, metabolic syndrome, and engagement in care, with promising initial findings of moderate improvements and engagement in health behaviors (Carrico & Moskowitz 2014; Celano et al 2018; Huffman et al 2015).

Research on PPIs will benefit from the inclusion of larger and more diverse clinical samples, and addressing broader outcomes, such as the impact of PPIs on resilience and healthy behaviors in primary care populations and patients with chronic diseases being treated in intensive LM settings. Though these interventions are still being refined and studied, there are many simple and practical ways that MPs can promote and study PP in clinical interactions.

Building the Evidence Base for Positive Psychology in Health Care

We need a strong evidence base to confidently translate these strategies into medical practice. Given several promising PP tools are emerging, we can recommend their use preliminarily. Further, collecting clinical practice data on the use of these PP strategies for outcomes such as well-being, mental health, and health behaviors and related outcomes will strengthen the translational evidence base. Involvement of the complete practice team will be essential in this type of translational research. A medical assistant can give a patient a screening tool, such as those introduced in Chapter 4, assessing self-reported positive affect, optimism, gratitude, and strengths, and input these scores into the medical record. The practitioner can follow up on these scores and use questions and statements like those suggested in Chapter 4 on clinic redesign to help improve total well-being. At follow-up visits, scores can be assessed again, and the process continued, modifying the PPI to overcome specific challenges as they arise. This approach would allow for longitudinal data collection on the effectiveness of these types of brief PPIs. Translational research thrives on implementation and iteration of interventions in "real world" settings.

Referrals to a mental health professional (e.g., social worker, psychologist) might be warranted when a patient demonstrates an adverse response to a PPI, such as increased depression symptoms or rumination about their lack of experienced positive emotions. Collaboration is warranted between non-mental health care and mental health care settings to identify best practices for referrals of such cases.

Because PPIs have been shown to improve psychological and subjective well-being and positive affect in the general population and in patients who do not meet criteria for a mental illness (as reviewed in Chapters 2 and 3), research on best practices for health care settings serving broad patient populations needs expansion. Moreover, with indications that these PP constructs are beneficial for improving quality of life for all individuals, patients and providers alike (see Chapter 9 on practitioner well-being), research to examine the impact of integrating these approaches for practitioner satisfaction and well-being is another essential topic. Important for PPI implementation and research in medical practices is the reduction of stigma associated with the term "positive psychology." Building the evidence and disseminating it may help counter the stigma and relay how these interventions have the potential to promote positive experiences and states of well-being, resilience and flourishing for anyone.

Gaps in Research on Positive Psychology for Health Care Settings

Two major gaps in research need to be addressed to advance the use of PPIs and tools in health care settings. The field's primary gap is the need to bridge the PPI research into mainstream clinical practice. Limited translational research is currently taking place. Inter-professional clinical teams who are open to using research-informed interventions can offer a solution. Practitioners can attend conferences on relevant topics for continuing education credits, which would also help bridge this gap. Embedded PP experts (e.g., trained psychologists, social workers, coaches) can implement research-informed interventions. Health care clinicians and PP researchers can collaborate to bring more interventions to practices.

Because the health care-PPI literature is an emerging field, the second gap is limited data available to suggest specific interventions for targeted outcomes in different populations. Therefore, simple strategies can be implemented at medical visits to help patients think more broadly about their strengths, optimism, gratitude, and positive affect. Healthcare teams can implement research-informed practices (practices identified in the psychology literature), in their settings as part of health action plans, and track outcomes. Such informal evaluation (described in Chapter 8) can be useful while the evidence-base for specific health care settings and populations is being built.

One key research area suggests that noticing and experiencing more positive emotions during health behaviors (e.g., physical activity, meditation) can increase a person's resources and motivation to continue this behavior (Van Cappellen et al 2018). To refine PPIs in support of health counseling and treatment plans, medical practitioners and PP researchers can tailor and test these positive activities for specific patients and practices. Referrals to health care team and counseling professionals who emphasize positive activities and prescriptions for relevant self-improvement digital apps can be evaluated for impact on health behaviors and long-term outcomes.

Examples of Translational Research Questions

To advance effective integration of PP approaches into health care practice, a number of research questions need to be answered. A few central questions for the field are:
1) Which specific PPIs can influence health and well-being outcomes, and for whom do they work?
2) Can we implement simple yet meaningful PP strategies into medical practices?
3) What is the feasibility and acceptability of clinical PP to patients and providers?
4) Do these PP strategies help with outcomes in real-world clinical settings related to mood, health related quality of life, health behaviors (diet, exercise, smoking cessation, medication adherence), stress management, and downstream disease outcomes?

Data Collection in Health Care Practices

Medical practitioners interested in participating in this translational research can collect data using the PP-based assessment tools that are integrated into care. Some examples are suggested in Chapter 4 and additional tools can be found in Chapter 12. Collection of such data from brief practical tools used during routine clinic intakes would provide insights into the impact of feasible strategies on outcomes. For efficiency in busy practices, some single-item screening measures using 0-10 Likert scale responses can be used.

To assess feasibility and acceptability of the clinical PPIs, patients could rate their experiences of ease and helpfulness on 0-10 scales. Medical records could be checked to assess medical outcomes of interest over time to determine whether relationships exist between the applied PPIs and outcomes.

Collaboration with Behavioral Medicine Researchers

Several strategies are recommended for collaboration between medical practitioners and behavioral medicine researchers. Partnerships between practitioners and researchers can solidify methods of data collection and work toward joint publications, which further increase the salience of PP. Medical practitioners can approach local universities' public health, psychology, or social work departments to suggest colleagues with whom to collaborate on translational research projects. Also, practitioners can partner with organizations like the Society of Behavioral Medicine (SBM), the International Positive Psychology Association (IPPA), the Positive Psychology Center at the University of Pennsylvania, the American Psychiatric or Psychological Associations (APAs), and the American Psychosomatic Society (APS) to promote and guide the design of PP translational research so the interventions studied are relevant, feasible, user-friendly and practical for health care practices. Practitioners interested in research can reach out to research partners to develop clear hypotheses and methods for collecting data and executing the interventions to be studied.

Coordination with Positive Psychology and Behavioral Medicine Research Communities

Opportunities are arising for medicine and health care innovation communities to coordinate and collaborate with professional PP and behavioral medicine societies such as SBM, IPPA, and other partners. Examples of research groups, academic health centers, health systems, and others active in PP for health that can provide resources and networking opportunities for research collaboration include:

- SBM's Scientific and Professional Liaison Council: https://www.sbm.org/about/leadership
- IPPA's research opportunities: https://www.ippanetwork.org/research/
- American Psychosomatic Society's Affect Science in Medicine group: https://www.psychosomatic.org
- Harvard T.H. Chan School of Public Health's Center for Health and Happiness: https://www.hsph.harvard.edu/health-happiness/
- The VA's Whole Health Initiative: https://www.va.gov/patientcenteredcare/explore/about-whole-health.asp
- UC Berkeley's Greater Good Science Center: https://greatergood.berkeley.edu/

Implementation of Current Positive Psychology Research

While medical practitioners with interest and opportunity to participate in this research begin to increase their involvement with it, other practitioners can champion and lead changes in their health care settings and organizations. As noted in Chapters 3 and 4, with guidance from research partners and an understanding of the current best research, practitioners can implement or prescribe simple, brief, approachable, acceptable, and effective PPIs. In larger health systems, practitioners can use the research to advocate for changes in the standard intakes and interventions, as well as model these changes in teaching programs. Chapter 10 discusses advocacy and teaching approaches.

High quality practical research, along with well-conducted meta-analyses, can be reviewed in order to adapt the lessons learned in medical practice. Meta-analyses are beneficial in offering succinct summaries of the PPIs studied. Medical practitioners can refer to these summaries to quickly identify PP research that has been done in specific populations, the type and setting of interventions used, and outcomes. Specific examples include:

- Sin & Lyubomirsky 2009: A meta-analysis of 51 interventions with 4,266 individuals concluded that PPIs should be offered for patient populations, especially those with mental health/mood disorders, older individuals, and those motivated to make well-being improvements. Individual interventions and those of longer duration may have greater impact than group or shorter interventions.
- Bolier et al. 2013: A meta-analysis of 39 studies and 6,138 participants showed that PPIs can improve subjective and psychological well-being and reduce depressive

symptoms. The authors encourage high quality clinical studies in diverse populations to strengthen the evidence base for PPIs.
- Chakhissi et al. 2018: A systemic review and meta-analysis of 30 studies and 1,864 patients showed small, but significant, effect sizes for well-being and depression compared to controls when omitting outliers. Significant moderate improvement of anxiety was also shown. These authors also noted the need for more, high quality studies.
- Kubzansky et al. 2018: Research of PPIs and cardiovascular health suggests that mindfulness-based programs and PPIs show promise in these populations for improving psychological well-being. Authors recommend further research of PPIs to test them across other settings, identify mechanisms of action between PPIs and health and well-being, and assess impact on outcomes.

Summary

Table 1 summarizes the key concepts about PP research for health care covered in this chapter.

Table 1: Positive Psychology (PP) Research for Health Care Settings

Topic	Summary
The current status of PP research in health care	- PP research has increased rapidly since the 1990s. - Positive psychology interventions (PPIs) have been shown to improve mood and affect. - Research on PPIs to promote health behaviors and disease outcomes is still in its early phases.
Research-informed ways to apply PP in health care/clinical settings	Medical practitioners can: - Ask patients targeted questions to emphasize PP constructs such as optimism, gratitude, positive affect, personal strengths, and finding meaning/purpose. - Support these PP constructs in clinical dialogues with patients. - Recommend research-supported or theoretically sound apps for home practice of PP activities.
Translational research to facilitate integration of PPIs and tools into health care	Medical practitioners and PP researchers can: - Attend cross-discipline conferences. Medical practitioners can: - Partner with research societies and local universities to identify hypotheses and research methods. - Refer to published meta-analyses to see the current scope of the PP research and relevance to populations in health care.

Translational research questions	• For whom do different PPIs work? • For which outcomes do different PPIs work?
Data collection in health care practices as clinical pilots	• Integrate PP measures into routine medical care and EMR. • Assess PP constructs at each visit using brief measures and conduct follow-ups for targeted processes and outcomes.
Implementation of current PP research	• Medical practitioners can direct discussions with patients toward PP constructs (e.g., optimism, gratitude, positive affect, personal strengths). • If meaningful and relevant to health goals, medical practitioners can suggest brief, targeted PPIs to strengthen patients' PP constructs (e.g., optimism, gratitude, positive affect, personal strengths).

References

Bolier L, Haverman M, Westerhof GJ, et al. Positive psychology interventions: a meta-analysis of randomized controlled studies. *BMC Public Health* 2013;13(1).

Carrico AW, Moskowitz JT. Positive affect promotes engagement in care after HIV diagnosis. *Health Psychol.* 2014;33(7):686-689.

Celano CM, Albanese AM, Millstein RA, et al. Optimizing a positive psychology intervention to promote health behaviors following an acute coronary syndrome. *Psychosom Med.* 2018:1.

Chakhssi F, Kraiss JT, Sommers-Spijkerman M, et al. The effect of positive psychology interventions on well-being and distress in clinical samples with psychiatric or somatic disorders: a systematic review and meta-analysis. *BMC Psychiat.* 2018;18(1).

Huffman JC, Dubois CM, Millstein RA, et al. Positive psychological interventions for patients with type 2 diabetes: rationale, theoretical model, and intervention development. *J Diabetes Res.* 2015;2015:1-18.

Kubzansky LD, Huffman JC, Boehm JK, et al. Positive psychological well-being and cardiovascular disease: JACC health promotion series. *J Am Coll Cardiol.* 2018;72(12):1382-1396.

Millstein RA, Park ER, Thorndike AN, et al. A qualitative study: How emotions influence physical activity and diet in metabolic syndrome patients. *Obesity Week,* Washington, DC, November 2017.

Seligman ME. *Authentic Happiness: Using the New Positive Psychology to Realize Your Potential for Lasting Fulfillment.* Chicago: Simon and Schuster, 2004.

Seligman MEP, Steen TA, Park N, et al. Positive psychology progress: Empirical validation of interventions. *Am Psychol.* 2005;60(5):410-421.

Sin NL, Lyubomirsky S. Enhancing well-being and alleviating depressive symptoms with positive psychology interventions: a practice-friendly meta-analysis. *J Clin Psychol.* 2009;65(5):467-487.

Van Cappellen P, Rice EL, Catalino LI, et al. Positive affective processes underlie positive health behavior change. *Psychol Health* 2018;33(1):77-97.

Additional Resources

Blevins D, Farmer MS, Edlund C, et al. Collaborative research between clinicians and researchers: a multiple case study of implementation. *Implementation Sci.* 2010;5(1).

Grenier J, Chomienne MH, Gaboury I, et al. Collaboration between family physicians and psychologists: What do family physicians know about psychologists" work? *Canad Fam Physician* 2008;54(2):232-233.

Howell RT, Kern ML, Lyubomirsky S. Health benefits: Meta-analytically determining the impact of well-being on objective health outcomes. *Health Psychol Rev.* 2007;1(1):83-136.

Nyström ME, Karltun J, Keller C, et al. Collaborative and partnership research for improvement of health and social services: researcher's experiences from 20 projects. *Health Res Policy Sy.* 2018;16(1).

Supper I, Catala O, Lustman M, et al. Interprofessional collaboration in primary health care: a review of facilitators and barriers perceived by involved actors. *J Publ Health.* 2015;37(4):716-27.

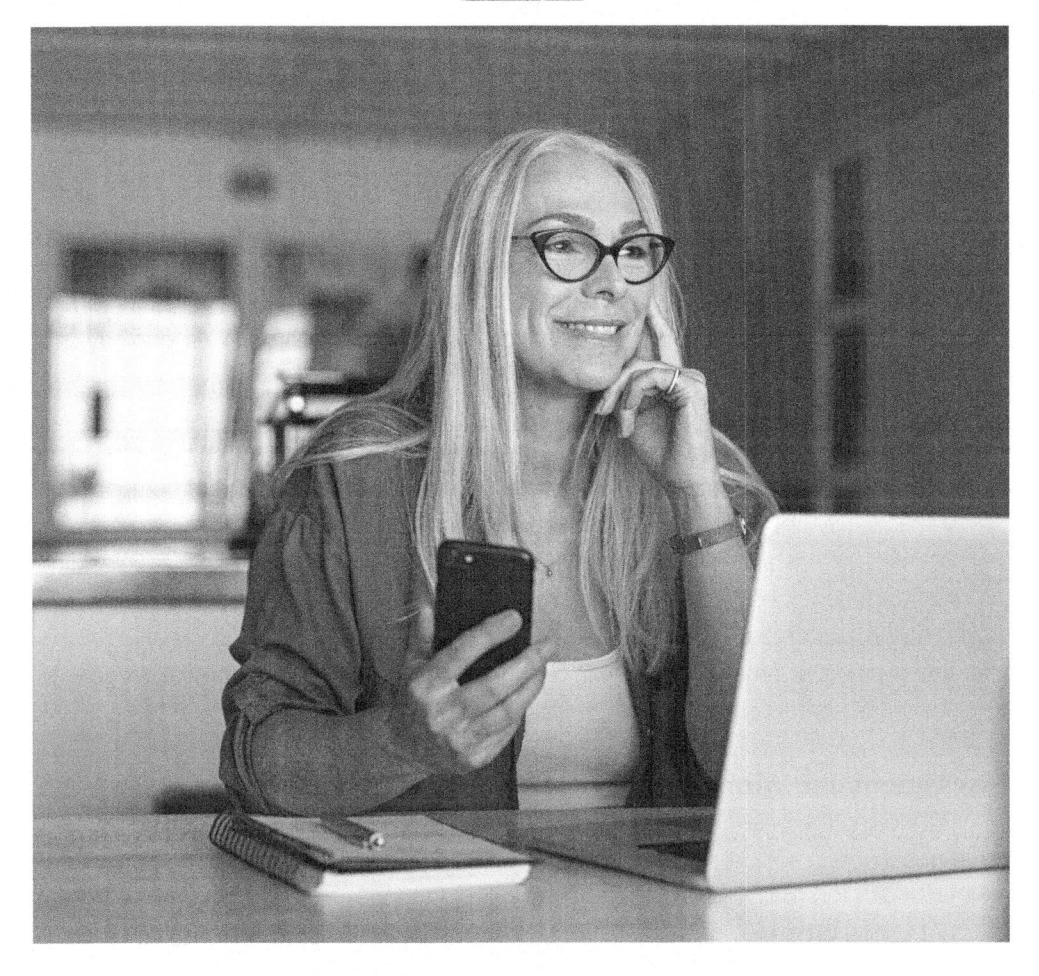

CHAPTER 12
Positive Psychology Resources
Janani Krishnaswami, Joe Raphael and Liana Lianov

Chapter Goal:
To assist health providers in efficiently and effectively implementing and prescribing positive psychology (PP) approaches through easy access tools and resources.

Chapter Highlights:
- Medical practitioners and health care teams can access a variety of assessment tools, scholarly and practical articles, books, and web resources to apply PP in health care practice.
- PP principles and strategies that can be adapted for health care settings are harnessed in smartphone applications and assessment and monitoring tools developed by some reputable groups.
- Resources from thought leaders in the field, reputable academic institutions and professional organizations offer guidance as this field expands research in areas relevant to health care.

Positive Psychology Tools and Resources

Lifestyle medicine practice and PP theories form a natural partnership. Emotional well-being is central to sustained behavioral transformation, including transitioning to whole-food plant-based nutrition, increasing physical activity, and prioritizing sleep. Emotional well-being is boosted by these health habits and through positive psychology interventions (PPIs) that cultivate the unique benefits of a healthy mindset. Two challenges that undermine application of PPIs are 1) lack of evidence on practical outcomes and applications in health care settings, and 2) low familiarity of medical practitioners and healthcare systems on how to apply PP tools developed and tested in psychology and behavioral health settings.

To complement the practical strategies for medical practitioners suggested in this handbook, this chapter offers guidance on available tools and resources. Such resources can facilitate the application of the theories of emerging PP research in personal and clinical practice. Multiple healthcare stakeholders, including clinical providers, community organizations, healthcare administrators, and research institutions can use the expanding research and resources to assist in scaling and translating theory into practice for improved health outcomes. We acknowledge that, due to the rapidly evolving nature of this field, the sources summarized here will change; we encourage the interested reader to conduct online searches for the latest releases and updates.

Assessment and Monitoring Tools and Resources

Choosing the best-fit measure and tool will depend on the amount of time or number of questions a medical setting's intake or vital sign process will accommodate. Moreover, choosing the tool will depend on the construct being measured; the main domains include positive emotions, life satisfaction, positive activities behaviors, and social connection. Chapter 4 provides an overview of happiness and emotional well-being assessment and monitoring tools. Healthy lifestyle tools are also essential for monitoring total well-being that impacts emotional well-being, but are beyond the scope of this handbook.

To conduct efficient initial assessments that can be included with screening the status of other health conditions and habits, medical practitioners can consider routine use of single item screening questions rated on a 1 to 10 Likert scale. Examples include:

- On a scale of 1-10, right now, how optimistic do you feel about your health?
- On a scale of 1-10, right now, how positive do you feel about the circumstances of your life?
- On a scale of 1-10, how grateful do you feel about your health?

For patients who score <5 on any of these screeners, follow up with relevant validated questionnaires can be considered, such as:

- The positive affect scale of the PANAS (Watson et al 1988)
- The LOT-R to measure optimism (Scheier et al 1994)
- The Gratitude Questionnaire--GQ-6 (McCullough et al 2001)
- The State Hope Scale (Snyder et al 1996)

We include in Table 1 examples of both proprietary and general domain tools. Sometimes permission is given for practitioners and researchers to use the proprietary or copyrighted tools. Please check the online information about permission for use or contact the developers of the measure. Many of these tools have been tested in psychology research settings and have yet to be tested in health care settings. Active champions of PP in health care might consider collaborating to test these measures in their health care settings. A number of these assessments can be taken online at https://authentichappiness.sas.upenn.edu/testcenter.

Table 1: Assessment and Monitoring Tools

Tool	Length	Study/ Reference	Web Link
Specific Trait Areas and Strengths			
Brief Strengths Scale	12 items, less than 10 minutes	Ho et al 2016	https://www.academia.edu/19549467/A_Brief_Strengths_Scale_for_Individuals_with_mental_health_issues
Gratitude Questionnaire	6 items, less than 5 minutes	McCullough et al 2002	https://ppc.sas.upenn.edu/resources/questionnaires-researchers/gratitude-questionnaire
GRIT Scale	10 items, 5 minutes	Duckworth & Quinn 2009; Duckworth et al 2007	https://angeladuckworth.com/grit-scale/
Life Orientation Test Revised: LOT-R Scale (optimism)	10 items 5 minutes	Scheier et al 1994	http://www.midss.org/content/life-orientation-test-revised-lot-r
Meaning in Life Questionnaire	10 items 5 minutes	Steger et al 2006	http://www.michaelfsteger.com/?page_id=13
Mindfulness Attention Awareness Scale	15 items 10 minutes	Brown & Ryan 2003	https://ppc.sas.upenn.edu/resources/questionnaires-researchers/mindful-attention-awareness-scale https://ggsc.berkeley.edu/images/uploads/The_Mindful_Attention_Awareness_Scale_-_Trait(1).pdf
Self-Compassion Scale – Short Form	12 items Less than 10 minutes	Raes et al 2011	www.self-compassion.org
Signature Strengths	120 items, less than 20 minutes	Peterson et al 2007	www.viacharacter.org
State Hope Scale	6 items, Less than 5 minutes	Snyder et al 1996	https://ppc.sas.upenn.edu/resources/questionnaires-researchers/adult-hope-scale

Table 1: Assessment and Monitoring Tools (continued)

General Happiness and Life Satisfaction			
Flourishing Scale	8 items, 5 minutes	Diener et al 2009	http://www.midss.org/content/flourishing-scale-fs-0 http://labs.psychology.illinois.edu/~ediener/FS.html https://ggsc.berkeley.edu/images/uploads/The_Flourishing_Scale.pdf
Oxford Happiness Questionnaire	29 items, 20 minutes	Hills & Argyle 2002	http://www.new.meaningandhappiness.com/oxford-happiness-questionnaire/214/
The PERMA Profiler	23 items, less than 20 minutes	Butler & Kern 2016	http://peggykern.org/uploads/5/6/6/7/56678211/the_perma-profiler_101416.pdf http://www.peggykern.org/questionnaires.html
Satisfaction with Life Scale (SWLS)	5 items, 2 minutes	Diener et al 1985; Pavot & Diener	http://www.midss.org/content/satisfaction-life-scale-swl
Skills-Based Happiness Quiz	14 items, less than 10 minutes	Based on the work of Ed Diener (Diener et al 1984, Diener 1994, Diener & Diener 1996)	www.pursuit-of-happiness.org
Subjective Happiness Scale	4 items, 2 minutes	Lyubomirsky & Lepper 1999	https:/sonjalyubomirsky.com/subjective-happiness-scale-shs/
Emotions			
Dispositional positive Emotion Scale (DPES)	38 items, 20 minutes	Shiota et al 2006	https://www.hsph.harvard.edu/health-happiness/dispositional-positive-emotion-scale/ http://wiki.mgto.org/doku.php/dispositional_positive_emotion_scale
PANAS Positive Affect and Negative Affect Schedule	20 items, 10 minutes	Watson et al 1988	https://www.toolshero.com/psychology/personal-happiness/panas-scale/

Profile of Mood Scale, shortened	24 to 40 items (different versions), less than 30 minutes	Morefield et al 2007; Grove & Prappavessis 1992; Shacham 1983	https://www.topendsports.com/psychology/poms.htm; https://www.researchgate.net/publication/299823508_Abrreviated_POMS_Questionaire_items_and_scoring_key
Positive Interactions			
Positivity Ratio	20 items, less than 15 minutes	Fredrickson 2013	www.positivityratio.com Note: The ratio is a guide (i.e. the higher, the better); but the Losada number of 3:1 has been criticized (Friedman 2018)

Resources for Positive Psychology Prescriptions

As introduced in Chapters 3 and 4, a simple way to begin incorporating PP into clinical practice is to prescribe regular positive activities, such as mindfulness or gratitude journaling. A variety of screening tools, questionnaires, and sample practices are also available for practitioners to use in selecting and developing positive psychology "prescriptions".

Web-Based Resources

The following list includes selected PP web-based resources with a variety of information including research summaries, articles, assessments, techniques and tips, and online communities.

- **Authentic Happiness** (https://www.authentichappiness.sas.upenn.edu/), operated by the University of Pennsylvania, has a series of questionnaires that are free to use with registration and can be administered to patients, staff, and providers.
- **Character Lab** (www.characterlab.com) contains a series of "playbooks" on various topics including gratitude, self-control, kindness, and grit; while geared at parents and teachers, these playbooks contain practical and actionable items that can be recommended for patients.
- The **Greater Good Science Center,** operated by University of California at Berkeley (https://greatergood.berkeley.edu/about), provides a clearinghouse of evidence-based practices, such as journaling techniques or meditation styles that can build positive character attributes, such as humility, calmness, kindness, and gratitude.
- The **Live Happy Magazine** (livehappy.com) offers a print and online publication, as well as podcasts, useful free articles, tips on positive living, and an online community that can be accessed by patients and providers.

Smartphone Applications

Overuse of social media and heavy smartphone use is increasingly recognized as a harbinger of isolation, inattention, scattered thinking, depression, and anxiety. However, smartphones may also represent a readily accessible, feasible format to help promote "default" healthy behavior for certain populations, including mindfulness and PP practice. While further research needs to be performed to solidify knowledge on outcomes, preliminary research suggests that web-based and smartphone-based applications can promote positive mood changes and behavioral outcomes (Lin et al 2018; Vandelanotte et al 2016). Focusing on these beneficial applications of smartphone use can help patients take the first step to improving habits and lifestyle. Many "apps" offer accessible ways for patients to sustain and reinforce positive psychology practices, such as mindfulness or gratitude, outside of the clinical setting. A selection of apps is presented in Table 2. Many have a free, light version with one exercise daily, with a paid option that unlocks a library of additional options and add-ons.

Table 2: Sample of Smartphone Application Resources

App Name	Description	Areas addressed
Calm	Secular approach to meditation that draws upon different cultures Guided meditations on a variety of topics, from self-esteem to managing emotions Soundscapes for focus and stress relief "Sleep Stories" for bedtime "Calm Body" movement practices to build physical health and resilience "Masterclasses" –in-depth class by experts on topics like mindful eating, building resilience, and sleep health	Meditation Stress reduction Insomnia Healthy habits Self-compassion Gratitude Physical movement
Happify	Offers various "tracks" customized to current life stressors and goals (input by user) Offers tracking tools to measure progress Clearinghouse of guided meditations Audio guides	
Headspace	Secular approach to meditation Guided meditations on a variety of topics, from self-esteem to managing emotions Bedtime and sleep stories Options for less guidance and free meditation Highly accessible for beginners, with classes on meditation basics Less focus on music and imagery	Meditation Stress reduction Insomnia Healthy habits Self-compassion Gratitude
Insight Timer	Clearinghouse of meditation practices from around the world (secular as well as drawing upon different world religions) Large offering of free meditations contributed by individuals around the world Also offers curated tracks and classes on different topics	Meditation Visualizations Tech-savvy meditator Looking to build own meditation practice More experienced meditator

Joyable	Offers a health coach and weekly assignments grounded in cognitive behavioral therapy, focusing on reduction of anxiety	Persons with generalized anxiety Stress management Looking for a personal coach/mentor
Shine	Offers daily text messages, articles, audio guides, and music to help address practical challenges of modern life Geared toward and led by women, but available to all	Women Workplace challenges Empathy and self-care

Resources for Building Knowledge

Building personal knowledge and familiarity with various dimensions of positive psychology is a good launch pad for considering making practice changes.

Thought Leaders in Positive Psychology

Review of the work of various thought leaders in the field is useful and enlightening. The following table (Table 3) presents a short (non-comprehensive) list of pioneers and thought leaders, several of whom have published books on their various subjects of expertise.

Table 3: Positive Psychology Thought Leadership Resources

Thought Leader	Focus Area	URL	Key Articles or Books
Mihaly Csikszentmihalyi	Flow	http://positivepsychology.org.uk/living-in-flow/	Csikszentmihalyi M. *Finding Flow. The Psychology of Engagement with Everyday Life.* New York: Basic Books, 1997.
Angela Duckworth	Grit, personality traits, success	https://angeladuckworth.com	Duckworth AL. Grit: *The Power of Passion and Perseverance.* New York: Simon and Schuster, 2016.
Sonja Lyubomirsky	Happiness, gratitude practice	http://sonjalyubomirsky.com	Lyubomirsky S. *The How of Happiness: A Scientific Approach to Getting the Life You Want.* New York, NY: The Penguin Press, 2008.
Martin Seligman	Flourishing and PERMA	https://www.authentichappiness.sas.upenn.edu	Seligman MEP. Flourish: *A Visionary New Understanding of Happiness and Well-Being.* New York, NY: Atria, 2011.

Ed Diener	Well-being: flourishing, life satisfaction	www.eddiener.com	Diener E, Diener RB. *Happiness: Unlocking the Mysteries of Psychological Wealth,* Blackwell: Oxford, 2008.
Barbara Fredrickson	Positive emotions, positivity ratio, positivity resonance, broaden-and-build theory, upward spiral of positive emotion	https://www.pursuit-of-happiness.org/history-of-happiness/barb-fredrickson/ https://www.positivityratio.com/single.php https://www.positvityresonance.com	Fredrickson BL. Positivity: *Top-Notch Research Reveals the Upward Spiral That Will Change Your Life.* New York: Three Rivers Press, 2009. Fredrickson B. Love 2.0: *Finding Happiness and Health in Moments of Connection.* New York: Plume, 2013.

Academic Institutions and Professional Organizations

Several academic and non-profit institutions offer informative, comprehensive websites that contain links to useful articles, seminal research, free tools, and grant opportunities, and serve as excellent launch pads for practitioners who are newer to the field of positive psychology. These include:
- **University of Pennsylvania – Positive Psychology Center**
- **Stanford University – Center for Altruism Research and Education**
- **Yale University – Center for Emotional Intelligence**
- **The Greater Good Science Center** – based at the University of California, Berkeley, but independently operated.

For advanced practitioners, opportunities also exist to obtain further training, degrees and certification in subfields of positive psychology. Examples include:
- **Benson Henry Institute** (Harvard University) – advanced training in stress management, resiliency and cognitive reappraisal training
- **Case Western Reserve University** – Certification in Organizational Management & Change
- **Stanford University** – Compassion Cultivation Training
- **University of Pennsylvania** – Online Foundations of Positive Psychology Specialization through Coursera
- **University of Pennsylvania** – Masters in Applied Positive Psychology

Other universities and centers that offer learning opportunities are listed in Table 4.

The **International Positive Psychology Association (IPPA),** the flagship membership organization for positive psychology worldwide, offers useful educational opportunities for health providers, especially through its Division of Positive Health and Wellness. The members of IPPA include practitioners and professionals from a variety of disciplines who work together to share and disseminate PP findings and research. The IPPA hosts its World Congress biannually and offers mentoring in PP. IPPA's learning library offers a wealth of resources, including recorded presentations from conferences, webinars, articles, and videos (https://www.ippanetwork.org/learninglibrary/).

Regional PP associations across the globe allow for networking and practice development through local collaboration and conferences. Additional organizations that offer membership and opportunities for collaboration with positive psychology experts include: the American Psychological Association (Division 38 – Society for Health Psychology; Division 47 – Society for Sport, Exercise and Performance Psychology) and the Society of Behavioral Medicine.

Several other organizations and stakeholders have also served as champions of PP and well-being in various domains. The following is a selected list of programs that incorporate PP techniques:

- **Veterans Health Administration – Whole Health for Life Program**
- **Stanford University – WELL for Life program**
- **Kaiser Permanente Medical Group – Thrive Campaign Program**
- **Massachusetts General Hospital Cardiac Psychiatry Program** – Offers PPIs for cardiovascular disease, diabetes mellitus, metabolic syndrome
- **HERO** – Health Enhancement Research Organization – Well-being scorecards

Table 4: Academic and Organizational Resources

University & Professional Associations	Center and/or Organizational Aim	URL	Training/Education Opportunities
American College of Lifestyle Medicine	Educating, equipping and empowering to prevent, treat, and reverse chronic disease	https://www.lifestyle-medicine.org/	Annual meeting, webinars, online training focused on lifestyle medicine, including PP
American Psychosomatic Society (APS)	Integrating mind, brain, body and social context into medicine	https://www.psychosomatic.org/home/index.cfm	Annual meeting, APS Journal
Case Western Reserve University	Organizational Behavior	https://www.coursera.org/casewesternreserve	Certification in organizational management and change
Claremont Graduate University	Division of Behavioral & Organizational Sciences	https://www.cgu.edu/academics/program/positive-health-psychology	Psychology program on optimism, physical health, positive health behaviors, social support/relationships to maximize health and well-being
Harvard University	Benson Henry Institute	www.bensonhenryinstitute.org	Advanced training in stress management, resiliency and cognitive reappraisal training
Health Enhancement Research Organization	Advancing health, well-being through employer leadership	https://hero-health.org/hero-scorecard/	Well-being scorecards

International Positive Psychology Association	Positive Psychology – research application, facilitate collaboration, share findings	https://www.ippanetwork.org/	Member access to a large library on positive psychology and health: https://www.ippa-network.org/learninglibrary
Society of Behavioral Medicine	Multi-specialty professionals improving health and quality of life through proven behavioral science	https://www.sbm.org/	Annual meeting and scientific sessions in behavioral medicine
Stanford University	Center for Altruism Research and Education	http://ccare.stanford.edu/	Compassion cultivation training WELL for Life program
University of Pennsylvania	Positive Psychology Center	www.ppc.sas.upenn.edu; https://www.coursera.org/specializations/positivepsychology	
University of California, Berkeley	Greater Good Science Center	https://greatergood.berkeley.edu/	Information and education on evidence-based practices addressing: community, culture, education, media & tech, mind & body, relationships, parenting & family, politics, spirituality, workplace
Yale University	Yale Center for Emotional Intelligence	http://ei.yale.edu/	Research and education: Emotions drive learning, decision-making, creativity, relationships, and health.
The Wholebeing Institute		https://wholebeinginstitute.com	Certificate in whole-being positive psychology (covering the science and direct application of PP); PP coaching certification

Additional Resources

A large variety of additional resources are available, including scientific articles, books, blogs, and assistance for local/community engagement. Selected examples are listed here.

Community Resource and Research Centers

- **Action for Happiness** (https://www.actionforhappiness.org), a movement led by Richard Layard and others in the United Kingdom, bringing together people from all walks of life, drawing on the latest scientific research, to take practical action in their communities to improve well-being.
- **Harvard Center for Health and Happiness** (https://www.hsps.harvard.edu/health-happiness) conducts research on a variety of topics related to positive psychology and well-being, such as the impact of positive emotions, forgiveness, optimism, green space, and technology on health and well-being.

Journals

- **The Journal of Positive Psychology**–peer reviewed journal covering positive psychology, optimism, resilience; aims to further research and promote good practice: https://www.tandfonline.com/toc/rpos20/current.
- **Journal of Positive Psychology and Well-Being**–peer reviewed academic journal that provides an interdisciplinary and international forum for the science of positive psychology and well-being: https://www.journalppw.com/index.php/JPPW.
- **Journal of Happiness Studies**–peer reviewed interdisciplinary scientific journal covering the study of happiness and well-being: https://link.springer.com/journal/10902.

Summary

A multitude of research-informed resources in the form of books, journals, scholarly articles, websites with summaries of key and recent studies, and digital apps are available to assist the physician and health care team interested in learning more about positive psychology and its contributing elements. Personal application of practical strategies to boost physician and health professional well-being and initiate an understanding of the benefits of these activities is highly recommended. As the practitioner becomes more familiar with key tools and resources, he or she will identify the best path for integrating these interventions into health care practice.

Selected Scientific Articles and Book Resources by Topic
Assessment

Brown KW, Ryan RM. The benefits of being present: Mindfulness and its role in psychological well-being. *J Pers Soc Psychol.* 2003;84:822-848.

Butler J, Kern M. The PERMA-Profiler: A brief multidimensional measure of flourishing. *Int J Well-Being* 2016;6(3):1-48.

Diener E. Measuring Subjective Well-being: Progress and opportunities. *Soc Indic Res.* 1994;28:35-89.

Diener E, Emmons RA, Larson RJ, et al. The satisfaction with life scale. *J Pers Assess.* 1985;49:71-75.

Diener E, Wirtz D, Tov W, et al. New measures of well-being: Flourishing and positive and negative feelings. *Soc Indic Res.* 2009;39:247-266.

Duckworth AL, Quinn PD. Development and validation of the Short Grit Scale (GritS). *J Pers Assess.* 2009; 91:166-174.

Fredrickson BL. Updated thinking on positivity ratios. *Am Psychol* 2013;68(9):814-822.

Friedman HL, Brown NJL. Implications of debunking the "critical positivity ratio" for humanistic psychology: Introduction to special issue. *J Humanist Psychol.* 2018;58(3):239-261

Grove JR, Prapavessis H. Preliminary evidence for the reliability and validity of an abbreviated Profile of Mood States. *Int J Sports Psychol.* 1992;23:93-109.

Hills P, Argyle M. The Oxford Happiness Questionnaire, A compact scale for the measurement of psychological well-being. *Pers Indiv Differ.* 2002;33(7):1073-1082.

Ho SMY, Li WL, Duan W, et al. A brief strengths scale for individuals with mental health issues. *Psychol Assess.* 2016;28(2):147.

Lopex SL, Snyder CR. Positive Psychological Assessment: *A Handbook of Models and Measures,* Washington DC: American Psychological Association Publishing, 2003.

Lyubomirsky S, Lepper HS. A measure of subjective happiness: Preliminary reliability and construct validation. *Soc Indic Res*. 1999; 46:137-155.

MacKillop J, Anderson EJ. Further psychometric validation of the Mindful Attention Awareness Scale (MAAS). *J Psychopathol Behav Access* 2007;29:289-293.

Morefield M, Petersen C, Bödeker AK, et al. The assessment of mood at workplace-psychometric analyses of the revised Profile of Mood States (POMS) questionnaire *Psychosoc Med*. 2007;4:Doc6.

Organization for Economic Co-operation and Development. Oxford Happiness Questionnaire, OECD Guidelines on Measuring Subjective Well-being, 2013.

Pavot W, Diener E. The Satisfaction with Life Scale and the emerging construct of life satisfaction. *J Posit Psychol*. 2008;3(2):137-152.

Raes F, Pommier E, Neff KD, et al. Construction and factorial validation of a short form of the self-compassion scale. *Clinl Psychol Psychoth*. 2010;18:250-255.

Shacham S. A shortened version of the Profile of Mood States. *J Pers Assess*. 1983;47(3):305-306.

Scheier MF, Carver CS, Bridges MW. Distinguishing optimism from neuroticism (and trait anxiety, self-mastery, and self-esteem): A reevaluation of the Life Orientation Test. *J Pers Soc Psychol*. 1994;67(6):1063-1078.

Steger MF, Frazier P, Oshi S, et al. The Meaning in Life Questionnaire: Assessing the presence of and search for meaning in life. *J Couns Psychol*. 2006;53:80-93.

Snyder CR, Sympson SC, Ybasco FC, et al. Development and validation of the State Hope Scale. *J Pers Soc Psychol*. 1996;70(2):321-335.

Watson D, Clark LA, Tellegen A. Development and validation of brief measures of positive and negative affect: The PANAS scales. *J Pers Soc Psychol*. 1988;54:1063-1070.

Character Strengths

Martinez-Marti ML, Ruch W. Character strengths predict resilience over and above positive affect, self-efficacy, optimism, social support, self-esteem, and life satisfaction. *J Posit Psychol*. 2017;12(2):110-119.

Niemiec RM. VIA Character Strengths-Research and Practice: The first ten years. In Knoop HH, Delle Fave A. (Eds). *Well-being and Cultures: Perspectives on Positive Psychology*, New York: Springer, 2013.

Park N, Peterson C. Character strengths: Research and practice. *J Coll Charact*. 2009; 10(4)

Peterson C, Ruch W, Beerman U, et al. Strengths of character, orientations to happiness, and life satisfaction. *J Posit Psychol*. 2007;2(3):149-156.

Peterson C, Seligman MEP. *Character Strengths and Virtues: A Handbook and Classification*. Washington, DC: American Psychological Association Press and Oxford University Press, 2004.

Digital Intervention Studies

Bolier L, Abello KM. Online positive psychological interventions: State of the art and future directions. In Parks AK, Schueller SM. (Eds), *The Wiley-Blackwell Handbook of Positive Psychological Interventions*. Oxfrod, England: Wiley-Backwell, 2014, p. 286-309.

Cobb NK, Poirier J. Effectiveness of a multimodal online well-being intervention: A randomized controlled trial. *Am J Prev Med*. 2013;46:41-41.

Lin Y, Tudor-Sfetea C, Siddiqui S, et al. Effective behavioral changes through a digital mhealth app: Exploring the impact of hedonic well-being, psychological empowerment and inspiration. *JMIR Mhealth Uhealth*, 2018;6(6): e10024.

Schueller SM, Parks AC. Disseminating self-help: Positive psychology exercises in an open online trial. *J Med Internet Res*. 2012;14:e63.

Vandelanotte C, Müller AM, Short CE. Past, present, and future of eHealth and mHealth research to improve physical activity and dietary behaviors. *J Nutr Educ Behav*. 2016;48(3):219-28.

General Positive Psychology Topics

Biswas-Diener R, Kashdan TB, Minhas G. A dynamic approach to psychological strength development and intervention. *J Posit Psychol*. 2011;6(2):106-118.

Brown B. *Rising Strong*, New York: Spiegel & Grau, Random House, 2015.

Brown FM, LaJambe CM. *Positive Psychology and Well-Being: Applications for Enhanced Living*. San Diego: Cognella Publ., University Readers, 2017.

Brown SL, Vaughan CC. *Play: How It Shapes the Brain, Opens the Imagination, and Invigorates the Soul*. New York: Avery, 2009.

Csikszentmihalyi M. *Finding Flow. The Psychology of Engagement with Everyday Life*. New York: Basic Books, 1997.

Diener E. Subjective Well-being. *Psychol Bull*. 1984;95:542-575.

Duckworth AL, Peterson C, Matthews MD, Kelly DR. Grit: Perseverance and passion for long-term goals. *J Pers Soc Psychol*. 2007;9:1087-1101.

Kubzansky LD, Huffman JC, Boehm JK, et al. Positive psychological well-being and cardiovascular disease: JACC health promotion series. *J Am Coll Cardiol*. 2018;72(12):1382-1396.

Lyubomirsky S. *The How of Happiness: A Scientific Approach to Getting the Life You Want*. New York, NY: The Penguin Press, 2008.

Oettingen G, Gollwitzer PM. Strategies of setting and implementing goals. In Maddux JD, Tangney JP (Eds.), *Social Psychological Foundations of Clinical Psychology*. New York, NY: The Guilford Press, 2010.

Seligman, MEP. *Flourish: A Visionary New Understanding of Happiness and Well-Being*. New York, NY: Atria, 2011.

Shiota MN, Keltner D, John OP. Positive emotion dispositions differentially associated with Big Five Personality and attachment style. *J Posit Psychol*. 2006;1(2):61-71.

Wong PTP. Positive psychology 2.0: Towards a balanced interactive model of the good life. *Canad Psychol*. 2011;52(2), 69-8.

Gratitude

Emmons RA. *Gratitude Works: A 21-Day Program for Creating Emotional Prosperity*. San Francisco, CA: Jossey-Bass. 2013.

McCullough ME, Emmons RA, Tsang J. The Grateful Disposition: A conceptual and Empirical Topography. *J Pers Soc Psychol*. 2002;82:112-127.

Grit

Duckworth AL. *Grit: The Power of Passion and Perseverance*. New York: Simon and Schuster, 2016.

Dweck CS. *Mindset: The New Psychology of Success*. New York: Ballantine Books, 2008.

Mindfulness

Beach MC, Roter D, Korthuis PT, et al. A multicenter study of physician mindfulness and health care quality. *Ann Fam Med*. 2012;11(5), 421-428.

Stahl B. Goldstein E, Santorelli S, Kabat-Zinn J. *A Mindfulness-Based Stress Reduction Workbook*. Oakland, CA: New Harbinger Publications, 2010.

Positive Emotion Studies and Scholarly Articles

Fredrickson BL. What good are positive emotions? *Rev Gen Psychol.* 1998;2:300-319.

Fredrickson BL. The role of positive emotions in positive psychology: The broaden-and-build theory of positive emotions. *Am Psychol.* 2001;56:218-226.

Fredrickson B. The broaden-and-build theory of positive emotions. *Philos Trans R Soc Lond B Biol Sci.* 2004; 359(1449):1367-1378.

Fredrickson BL, Tugade MM, Waugh CE, et al. What good are positive emotions in crisis? *J Pers Soc Psychol.* 2003;84(2):365-376.

Fredrickson BL, Cohn MS, Coffey KA, et al. Open hearts build lives: Positive emotions, induced through loving-kindness meditation, build consequential personal resources. *J Pers Soc Psychol.* 2008;95(5):1045-1062.

Kubzansky LD, Thurston R. Emotional vitality and incident coronary heart disease. *Arch Gen Psychiat.* 2007;64: 1393–1401.

Stellar JE, John-Henderson N, Anderson CL, et al. Positive affect and markers of inflammation: discrete positive emotions predict lower levels of inflammatory cytokines. *Emotion* 2015;15(2):129-33.

Social Connection

Sandstrom GM, Dunn EW. Social interactions and well-being: The surprising power of weak ties. *Pers Soc Psychol B.* 2014;40:910-922.

Valliant GE. *Aging well: Surprising Guideposts to a Happier Life from the Landmark Harvard Study of Adult Development*. Boston, MA: Little, Brown, 2002.

Alpha Listing of Web Resources (Noted in Tables of this Chapter)

Action for Happiness: https://www.actionforhappiness.org

American College of Lifestyle Medicine: https://www.lifestylemedicine.org/

Benson Henry Institute: www.bensonhenryinstitute.org

Cigna Health: https://wellbeing.cigna.com

Diener, Edward. ENHANCE program and other resources: www.eddiener.com

The Gallup Strengths Center: https://www/gallup.com/cliftonstrengths/en/home/aspx

Greater Good in Action: https://ggia.berkeley.edu

Greater Good Science Center: https://greater.good.berkely.edu

Harvard Center for Happiness and Health, TH Chan School of Public Health: https://www.hsph.harvard.edu/health-happiness

International Positive Psychology Association: https://www.ippanetwork.org/

Journal of Positive Psychology and Well-Being: https://www.journalppw.com/index.php/JPPW

Kaiser Permanente Program: https://thrive.kaiserpermanente.org/

Live Happy Magazine: https.//www.livehappy.org

Massachusetts General Cardiac Psychiatry Program: https://www.massgeneral.org/Psychiatry/Research/researchlab.aspx?id=1829

Masters in Applied Postive Psychology: https://www.sas.upenn.edu/lps/graduate/mapp

Mayo Clinic Healthy Living Program: https://healthyliving.mayoclinic.org

Society of Behavioral Medicine: www.sbm.org

Positive Psychology Center: https://ppc.sas.upenn.edu

Pursuit of Happiness site with Happiness Skills Quiz: https://www.pursuit-of-happiness.org

The Journal of Positive Psychology: https://www.tandfonline.com/toc/rpos20/current

Veterans Health Administration – Whole Health for Life Program: https://www.va.gov/patientcenteredcare/explore/about-whole-health.asp

Signature Strengths/Virtues in Action: VIA Institute on Character. VIA Character Survey: https://www.viacharacter.org

The Wholebeing Institute: https://wholebeinginstitute.com

References (Cited in Chapter Text)

Brown KW, Ryan RM. The benefits of being present: Mindfulness and its role in psychological well-being. *J Pers Soc Psychol.* 2003;84:822-848.

Butler J, Kern M. The PERMA-Profiler: A brief multidimensional measure of flourishing. *Int J Well-Being* 2016;6(3):1-48.

Diener E. Measuring Subjective Well-being: Progress and opportunities. *Soc Indic Res.* 1994;28:35-89.

Diener E, Emmons RA, Larson RJ, et al. The satisfaction with life scale. *J Pers Assess.* 1985;49:71-75.

Diener E, Diener C. Most people are happy. *Psychol Sci,* 1996;7(3):181-185.

Diener E, Wirtz D, Tov W, et al. New measures of well-being: Flourishing and positive and negative feelings. *Soc Indic Res.* 2009;39:247-266.

Duckworth AL, Peterson C, Mathews MD, et al. Grit: Perseverance and passion for long-term goals. *J Pers Soc Psychol.* 2007;92(6):1087-1101.

Duckworth AL, Quinn PD. Development and validation of the Short Grit Scale (GritS). *J Pers Assess.* 2009; 91:166-174.

Fredrickson BL. Updated thinking on positivity ratios. *Am Psychol* 2013;68(9):814-822.

Grove JR, Prapavessis H. Preliminary evidence for the reliability and validity of an abbreviated Profile of Mood States. *Int J Sports Psychol.* 1992;23:93-109.

Hills P, Argyle M. The Oxford Happiness Questionnaire Aa compact scale for the measurement of psychological well-being. *Pers Indiv Differ.* 2002;33(7):1073-1082.

Ho SMY, Li WL, Duan W, et al. A brief strengths scale for individuals with mental health issues. *Psychol Assess.* 2016;28(2):147.

Lin Y, Tudor-Sfetea C, Siddiqui S, et al. Effective behavioral changes through a digital mhealth app: Exploring the impact of hedonic well-being, psychological empowerment and inspiration. *JMIR Mhealth Uhealth*, 2018;6(6): e10024.

Lyubomirsky S, Lepper HS. A measure of subjective happiness: Preliminary reliability and construct validation. *Soc Indic Res*. 1999; 46:137-155.

McCullough ME, Emmons RA, Tsang JA. The grateful disposition: A conceptual and empirical topography. *J Pers Soc Psychol.* 2002;82(1):112-127.

Morefield M, Petersen C, Bödeker AK, et al. The assessment of mood at workplace-psychometric analyses of the revised Profile of Mood States (POMS) questionnaire *Psychosoc Med.* 2007;4:Doc6.

Peterson C, Ruch W, Beerman U, et al. Strengths of character, orientations to happiness, and life satisfaction. *J Posit Psychol.* 2007;2(3):149-156.

Raes F, Pommier E, Neff KD, et al. Construction and factorial validation of short form of the Self-Compassion Scale. *Clin Psychol Psychot*. 2011(18):250-255.

Scheier MF, Carver CS, Bridges MW. Distinguishing optimism from neuroticism (and trait anxiety, self-mastery, and self-esteem): A reevaulation of the Life Orientation Test. *J Pers Soc Psychol*.1994;67(6):1063-1078.

Shacham S. A shortened version of the Profile of Mood States. *J Pers Assess*. 1983;47(3):305-306.

Shiota MN, Keltner D, John OP. Positive emotion dispositions differentially associated with Big Five Personality and attachment style. *J Posit Psychol*. 2006;1(2):61-71.

Snyder CR, Sympson SC, Ybasco FC, et al. Development and validation of the State Hope Scale. *J Pers Soc Psychol*. 1996;70(2):321-335.

Steger MF, Frazier P, Oshi S, et al. The Meaning in Life Questionnaire: Assessing the presence of and search for meaning in life. *J Couns Psychol*. 2006;53:80-93.

Vandelanotte C, Müller AM, Short CE. Past, present, and future of eHealth and mHealth research to improve physical activity and dietary behaviors. *J Nutr Educ Behav*. 2016;48(3):219-28.

Watson D, Clark LA, Tellegen A. Development and validation of brief measures of positive and negative affect: The PANAS scales. *J Pers Soc Psychol*. 1988;54:1063-1070.

Epilogue
Planning the Way Forward Orienting Medical Practice to Implement Positive Psychology
Liana Lianov

In this handbook, we highlight the reinforcing nature of lifestyle medicine (LM) and positive psychology (PP). We make the case that medical practitioners who aim to promote total well-being should consider addressing the element of positive health as a standard in lifestyle medicine and primary care. Other medical specialists and health professionals who emphasize lifestyle interventions in their clinical practices will also find benefits from adding PP principles and interventions into routine care. This enhancement has the potential to drive health behavior change, induce physiologic benefits directly, and boost health outcomes.

Health care practices can promote total well-being by:
- Assessing emotional well-being and recommending positive activities for their patients
- Increasing positive interactions with patients and the health team
- Orienting health behavior coaching towards positive life goals
- Encouraging patients to implement positive activities into their well-being plans
- Applying principles of PP for physicians' and health professionals' self-care
- Engaging in translational research or partnering with researchers when feasible to grow the evidence base and build best practices for PP implementation in health care settings
- Teaching students and residents the principles of PP as part of routine care
- Advocating for system changes that support total well-being of patients and health providers

These actions not only have the potential to improve the well-being of patients, but also the well-being of physicians, other medical practitioners, and the entire health care team. Such changes are critical at a time when physician burn out and suicides are at high levels. Table 1 walks through the steps and questions to consider when making the shift to emphasize PP principles and interventions into a health care practice.

The recommendations provided in the handbook can assist practitioners to take these kinds of steps. Of course, it must be acknowledged that inadequate insurance coverage or reimbursement challenges the capacity of medical practitioners to spend adequate time with patients and tackle all pillars of total well-being. Yet, even brief interventions and referrals to outside resources are worth considering for achieving health outcomes. The need for scientific research to build the evidence base specifically for health care settings and to inform best practices is another challenge.

Despite these challenges, we hope that more medical practitioners will choose to implement some PP practices based on the psychological scientific literature for both their patients and themselves. We encourage you to advocate for the health care community to address total well-being (physical, mental, emotional, social, and positive health) and participate or collaborate with PP researchers to build the evidence base and best practice guidelines for future generations of practitioners.

Table 1: Integrating Positive Psychology (PP) Strategies into Practice

Key Steps	Prompts for Your Clinical Practice
Advocate/negotiate with health care leadership to emphasize total well-being, including positive psychology interventions (PPIs) as healthy lifestyle habits	Who are the decision makers? Who will lead this practice change? What is the near term opportunity to discuss this change? What scholarly evidence and research summaries do you need to make the case for a change? What is the motivation for the change, i.e., what goals would you like to achieve for the clinic? • Engage patients in health behavior change? Improve outcomes? • Boost health team and patient morale? Advance the clinic processes into innovative models of care? • Participate in research?
Choose a well-being assessment/measure(s)	Which measure(s) fit the practice change goal? Are you considering a small practice change? Are you already moving in this direction as a practice and aim to expand your capacity to assess and promote well-being? (These answers can guide appropriate length of the measure/assessments.)
Review and make changes to current assessment procedures and forms to add PP and well-being measure(s)	What assessment form(s) will you expand? • Initial encounter pre-assessment? • Standard check-in for all encounters? Will you make changes in virtual and/or hard copy assessments?
Review and identify online and local community resources that promote well-being	What community-based organizations in your area offer and/or support positive activities? What digital/technology access does your patient population have?

Determine special considerations for your patient population	What is the cultural background of the majority of your patient population? How could the culture of your patient population impact PPI results and require adjustments? Which types of PPIs would be most appropriate for your patient population? What is the socioeconomic status of your population? What can you offer to low income patients, e.g., instructions for simple mindfulness exercise, time in nature/sunshine, social connection?
Identify/list key positive activities to include in patient recommendations	How will you address positive health and PPIs in your practice? Which health team members will be designated to discuss the activities with patients or make referrals (with brief reinforcement from the practitioner)?
Engage and train the health care team	What are the opinions of your health care team about the change? What are their needs? Is there health care worker burnout that can be addressed by encouraging them to apply PPIs? What kind of training will work best (e.g., staff meeting, online-webinar training, intensive retreat)?
Change the health care culture and environment to embrace PP principles	What small changes can the health care team make to increase positive interactions within the team and with patients?
Conduct and evaluate a trial period of making a practice change to incorporate PP approaches	What evaluation measures, such as increased time spent with patients and health team and patient satisfaction levels, will you set? Who will conduct the evaluation after the trial period is completed, and how? What are the results that will be considered a success?
Implement the PP-related practice change and continue to improve it through a continuous quality improvement (CQI) process	Who is the CQI lead for this practice change(s)? How will this practice change be tracked over time?
Apply PP practices for the practitioner's personal well-being	Which elements of positive psychology and which positive activities are relevant to my personal life and professional career? What actions am I read to take now to improve my total well-being? How can I be a role model for my colleagues and patients?

Appendix A
PERMA Model
(Flourish by Martin Seligman)

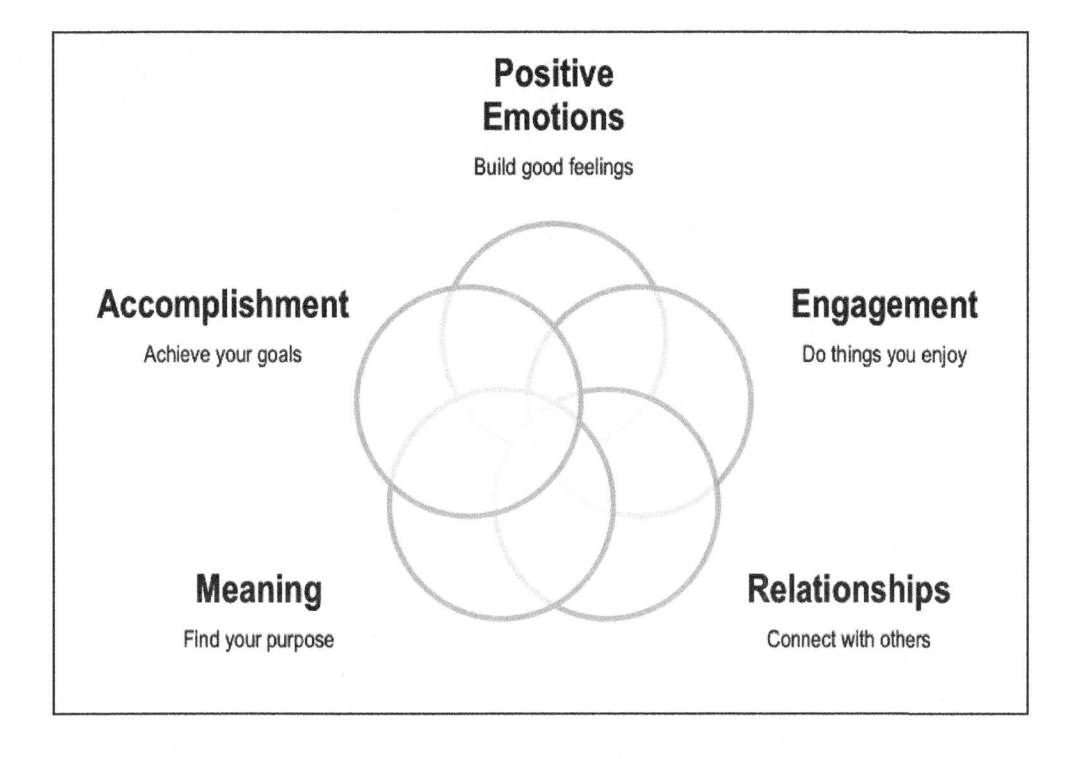

Positive Emotions
Build good feelings

Accomplishment
Achieve your goals

Engagement
Do things you enjoy

Meaning
Find your purpose

Relationships
Connect with others

Adapted from: Seligman M. *Flourish: A Visionary New Understanding of Happiness and Well-being*. New York: Free Press, 2011.

Appendix B:
Summary of Key Positive Psychology Interventions

Practice	Physiologic/Health Effects	Intervention
Meditation	• Interoceptive awareness of bodily and emotional states (Magalhaes et al 2018) • Signal decreases in the amygdala (Lazar 2000) • Lower self-reported stress intensity by 26% (Engert et al 2017) • The vagal nerve, as a proponent of the parasympathetic nervous system (PNS), is the prime candidate for explaining the effects of contemplative practices on physical and mental health and cognition (Gerritsen et al 2018)	• Breathing meditation • Body scan
Mindfulness	• Reduces anxiety and depression, manages physical pain symptoms, supports substance abuse recovery, and promotes well-being (Creswell 2017; Goldberg et al 2018) • Reduces negative affect and heart rate while increasing mood (Zeidan et al 2010)	• Paying attention to present-moment experience, on purpose, with an attitude of acceptance or non-judgment • Main techniques: awareness of breath, awareness of body sensations, walking meditation, and mindful movement, mindfulness based stress reduction (MBSR), mindfulness based cognitive behavioral therapy (MBCBT)

Loving kindness meditation (LMK)	• May enhance activation of brain areas that are involved in emotional processing and empathy (Hutcherson et al 2008) • Produces higher positive affect and more positive explicit and implicit evaluations of others (Hutcherson et al 2008) • May reduce depressive symptoms and increase positive emotions (Shahar et al 2015)	• Meditative exercise of unconditional kindness to address social anxiety, marital conflict, anger, and coping with the strains of long-term caregiving (Hofmann et al 2011) • Meditative exercise of unconditional kindness for immediate, daily positive emotions
Compassion	• Greater altruistic behavior may emerge from increased engagement in neural systems implicated in understanding the suffering of others, executive and emotional control, and reward processing (Weng et al 2013) • Reduces factors like rumination and self-criticism, but also improves positive mental health by enhancing factors such as kindness and positive emotions (Trompetter et al 2017) • May reduce stress-induced subjective distress and immune response (Trompetter et al 2017)	• Self-compassion meditation • Metta meditation
Gratitude	• When conducted regularly, such as writing down three good things in one's life, is shown to elicit heightened well-being across several outcomes measure, with the effect on positive affect as the most robust finding (Emmons & McCullough 2003) • Builds psychological, social and spiritual resources, aligned with the broaden and build model to developing enduring personal resources (Fredrickson 1998)	• Intervention of counting blessings or expressing gratitude

Positive activities	• Promote well-being by boosting positive emotions, thoughts, and behaviors, and need satisfaction (Lyubomirsky & Layous 2013) • Reduce rumination and loneliness and allow for adaptive coping from environmental stressors (Layous et al 2013)	• Doing physical and mental activities that enhance energy and well-being
Flow	• The matched balance of perceived challenge and personal skills lead to optimal experience (Csikszentmihalyi & Csikszentmihalyi 1988)	• Seeking opportunities for actions in the surrounding environment that match the individual's abilities (Csikszentmihalyi & Csikszentmihalyi 1988) Flow Components: 1) Engaging in an activity that contains a clear set of goals that add direction and purpose/meaning to behavior 2) a balance between perceived challenges and perceived skills 3) the presence of clear and immediate feedback (Csikszentmihalyi & Csikszentmihalyi 1988)
Social connection	• ReSource Project: Psychosocial stress is reduced after long-term mental training in a broadly accessible low-cost approach to acquiring resilience (Engert et al 2017) • Social support impacts hypothalamic-pituitary-adrenocortical and noradrenergic systems and central oxytocin pathways (Ozbay et al 2007) • Micro-moments of connectivity improve vagal tone and increase heart rate variability (Fredrickson 2013)	• Short daily intersubjective (social interaction) practice • Inquiring about quantity and quality of social interactions and exploring methods for increasing brief social interactions and social support connections

Meaning and purpose	• Positive influence on biological, psychological and behavioral outcomes and may play an important role in protecting against heart disease in those at risk (Kim et al 2013) • Greater use of several preventive health care services and fewer nights spent hospitalized (Kim et al 2014)	• Exploring an individual's sense of directedness and sense of meaning in his or her life
Religion and spirituality	• Correlated with decreased mortality rates among healthy samples, even after controlling for potentially confounding behaviors (Chida et al 2009)	• Identifying involvement in religious or spiritual practice or community

References

Chida Y, Steptoe A, Powell, LH. Religiosity/spirituality and morality: A systematic quantitative review. *Psychoth Psychosom.* 2009;78:81–90.

Creswell JD. Mindfulness interventions. *Ann Rev Psychol.* 2017;68:491–516.

Csikszentmihalyi M, Csikszentmihalyi IS. *Optimal Experience: Psychological Studies of Flow in Consciousness.* New York: Cambridge University Press, 1988.

Emmons RA, McCullough ME. Counting blessings versus burdens: Experimental studies of gratitude and subjective well-being. *J Pers Soc Psychol.* 2003;84.2: 377-389.

Engert V, Ko BE, Papassotiriou, et al. Specific reduction in cortisol stress reactivity after social but not attention-based mental training. *Sci Adv.* 2017;3(10):e1700495.

Fredrickson BL. What good are positive emotions? *Rev Gen Psychol.* 1998;2(3):300-319.

Fredrickson BL. *Love 2.0.* New York City, NY: Plume, 2013.

Gerritsen R, Sebastiaan J, Band GPH. Breath of life: the respiratory vagal stimulation model of contemplative activity. *Front Hum Neurosci.* 2018;12:397.

Goldberg SB, Tucker RP, Greene PA, et al. Mindfulness-based interventions for psychiatric disorders: A systematic review and meta-analysis. *Clin Psychol Rev.* 2018;59:52–60.

Hofmann SG, Grossman P, Hinton E. Loving-kindness and compassion meditation: potential for psychological interventions. *Clin Psychol Rev.* 2011;31(7):1126-32.

Hutcherson CA, Seppälä EM, Gross JJ. Loving-kindness meditation increases social connectedness. *Emotion* 2008;8(5):720–4.

Kim ES, Sun JK, Park N, et al. Purpose in life and reduced risk of myocardial infarction among older US adults with coronary heart disease: a two-year follow-up. *J Behav Med.* 2013;36(2), 124-133.

Kim ES, Strecher VJ, Ryff CD. Purpose in life and use of preventive health care services. *Proc Natl Acad Sci.* 2014;111(46):16331-16336.

Layous K, Chancellor J, Lyubomirsky S. Positive activities as protective factors against mental;

health conditions. *J Abnorm Psychol.* 2013;123:2-12.

Lazar SW, Bush G, Gollub RL, et al. Functional brain mapping of the relaxation response and meditation. *Neuroreport* 2000;11(7):1581-1585.

Lyubomirsky Sonja, Layous K. How do simple positive activities increase well-being?. *Curr Dir Psychol Sci.* 2013;22(1):57-62.

Magalhaes AA, Oliveira L, Pereira MG, et al. Does meditation alter brain responses to negative stimuli? A systematic review. *Front Hum Neurosci.* 2018;12:448.

Ozbay F, Johnson DC, Dimoulas E, et al. Social support and resilience to stress. *Neurobiol Clin Pract.* 2007;4(5):35-40.

Piedmont RL. Does spirituality represent the sixth factor of personality? Spiritual transcendence and the five-factor model. *J Pers.* 1999;67, 985–1013.

Shahar B. Szepsenwol O, Zilcha-Mano S, et al. A wait-list randomized controlled trial of loving-kindness meditation programme for self-criticism. *Clin Psychol Psychot.* 2015;22(4):346-356.

Trompetter HR, de Kleine E, Bohlmeijer ET. Why does positive mental health buffer against psychopathology? An exploratory study on self-compassion as a resilience mechanism and adaptive emotion regulation strategy. *Cognitive Ther Res.* 2017;41(3):459-468.

Weng HY, Fox AS, Shackman AJ, et al. Compassion training alters altruism and neural responses to suffering. *Psychol Sci.* 2013;24(7):1171-1180.

Zeidan F, Johnson SK, Gordon NS, et al. Effects of brief and sham mindfulness meditation on mood and cardiovascular variables. *J Altern Complem Med.* 2010;16(8):867–73.

Appendix C:
Emotional Well-Being Assessment Tools

This appendix offers several commonly used, brief emotional well-being assessment tools. A health care setting may choose to use one or more of these assessments during clinic intakes and total well-being assessments, and while monitoring progress in improving emotional well-being. Please check online about rights to use each of these assessments for commercial purposes.

Patient Health Questionnaire 4

Feelings	Not at all	Several days	More days than not	Nearly every day
Feeling nervous, anxious or on edge	0	1	2	3
Not being able to stop or control worrying	0	1	2	3
Feeling down, depressed or hopeless	0	1	2	3
Little interest or pleasure in doing things	0	1	2	3

Total score = adding the scores for the 4 items: Normal (0-2), Mild (3-5), Moderate (6-8), Severe (9-12).

Assess anyone with a positive screen (mild, moderate or severe) for suicidal ideation.

A positive screen: follow-up with Patient Health Questionnaire (PHQ-9), the Hamilton Depression Scale [HAM-D] or other instruments.

Review *Diagnostic and Statistical Manual of Mental Disorders* criteria to establish a diagnosis and initiate a treatment/follow-up plan.

Kroenke K, Spitzer RL. An ultra-brief screening scale for anxiety and depression: The PHQ-4. *Psychosom*. 2009;50(6):613-621.

Adult Hope Scale

Using the scale below, select the number that best describes you and place it in the space.

1 = Definitely false
2 = Mostly false
3 = Somewhat false
4 = Slightly false
5 = Slightly true
6 = Somewhat true
7 = Mostly true
8 = Definitely true

___1. I can think of many ways to get out of a jam.

___2. I energetically pursue my goals.

___3. I feel tired most of the time.

___4. There are lots of ways around a problem.

___5. I am easily downed in an argument.

___6. I can think of many ways to get the things in life that are important to me.

___7. I worry about my health.

___8. Even when others get discouraged, I know I can find a way to solve the problem.

___9. My past experiences have prepared me well for my future.

___10. I've been pretty successful in my life.

___11. I usually find myself worrying about something.

___12. I meet the goals that I set for myself.

The agency subscale score is derived by adding 2, 9, 10, 12; the pathway subscale score is derived by adding 1, 4, 6, and 8. The total Hope Score is derived by summing the agency and pathway scores.

Snyder CR, Harris C, Anderson JR, et al. The will and the ways: Development and validation of an individual-differences measure of hope. *J Pers Soc Psychol. 1991;60:570-585.*

Flourishing Scale
(eddiener.com)

Below are 8 statements with which you may agree or disagree. Using the 1-7 scale below, indicate your agreement with each item by indicating that response for each statement.

1 = Strongly disagree
2 = Disagree
3 = Slightly disagree
4 = Mixed or neither agree nor disagree
5 = Slightly agree
6 = Agree
7 = Strongly agree

____ I lead a purposeful and meaningful life.

____ My social relationships are supportive and rewarding.

____ I am engaged and interested in my daily activities.

____ I actively contribute to the happiness and well-being of others.

____ I am competent and capable in the activities that are important to me.

____ I am a good person and live a good life.

____ I am optimistic about my future.

____ People respect me.

Diener E, Wetz D, Trov W, et al. New measures of well-being: Flourishing and positive and negative feelings. *Soc Indic Res*. 2009;99:247-266.

Schotanus-Dijkstra M, Klooster PM ten, Drossaert CHC, et al. Validation of the Flourishing Scale in a sample of people with suboptimal levels of mental well-being. *BMC Psychol*. 2016;4:12.

Satisfaction with Life Scale (SWLS)

Ed Diener's research suggests that the SWLS (for which the respondent rates the 5 items listed below on a seven point Liktert scale) has a significant correlation with health and longevity. In settings where shorter screens are needed, Diener recommends asking the two bolded items (Diener E. American College of Lifestyle Medicine Summit on Happiness Science in Health Care, 2018).

Below are five statements with which you may agree or disagree. Using the 1-7 scale below, indicate your agreement with each item by placing the appropriate number on the line preceding the item.

1 = strongly disagree
2 = disagree
3 = slightly disagree
4 = neither agree nor disagree
5 = slightly agree
6 = agree
7 = strongly agree

____ In most ways my life is close to my ideal.

____ The conditions of my life are excellent.

____ I am satisfied with my life.

____ So far I have gotten the important things I want in life.

____ If I could live my life over, I would change almost nothing.

Diener E, Emmons RA, Larsen RJ, Griffin S. The Satisfaction with Life Scale. *J Pers Assess.* 1985;48(1):71-75.

Subjective Happiness Scale

For each of the following statements and/or questions, please circle the point on the scale that you feel is most appropriate in describing you.

In general, I consider myself:

1	2	3	4	5	6	7
not a very happy person						a very happy person

Compared to most of my peers, I consider myself:

1	2	3	4	5	6	7
less happy						more happy

Some people are generally very happy. They enjoy life regardless of what is going on, getting the most out of everything. To what extent does this characterization describe you?

1	2	3	4	5	6	7
not at all						a great deal

Some people are generally not very happy. Although they are not depressed, they never seem as happy as they might be. To what extent does this characterization describe you?

1	2	3	4	5	6	7
not at all						a great deal

Item #4 is reverse coded.

Lyubomirsky S, Lepper H. A measure of subjective happiness: Preliminary reliability and construct validation. *Soc Indic Res.* 1999;46:137-155.

Appendix D
Identify and Use Your Strengths

Using your strengths makes it easier for you to achieve your goals.
- Circle your top 5-10 strengths from the list below or list your own.
- Decide what goal you want to achieve.
- Then pick the top strength or two that you'll use to help you achieve it.

Adaptable	Enthusiastic	Insightful	Persistent
Articulate	Efficient	Intuitive	Polite
Brave	Empathetic	Kind	Pro-active
Candid	Fair	Leader	Realistic
Cooperative	Flexible	Learner	Responsible
Creative	Forgiving	Loving	Responsive
Curious	Focused	Logical	Resourceful
Calm	Funny	Methodical	Sociable
Charismatic	Grateful	Open-minded	Self-directed
Considerate	Honest	Organized	Self-disciplined
Compassionate	Hopeful	Passionate	Spiritual
Competitive	Hard-working	Patient	Sensible
Decisive	Helpful	Perceptive	Sincere
Determined	Honest	Persuasive	Thoughtful
Diligent	Humble	Prudent	Thorough
Energetic	Innovative	Practical	Teamwork

Appendix E
Using Personality to Guide Selection of Positive Psychology Interventions

For Medical Practitioners: Overview of Personality Assessment and Guidance for Use

Carl Jung identified eight cognitive functions that guide how we view and interact with the world (Andrews 2014; Beebe 2013). The theory suggests that individuals with different personality types are comfortable with different thought processes. The Myers Briggs Personality Type Indicator (MBTI), which was subsequently developed by Myers and Briggs, is a widely used assessment tool for this personality framework. The psychometrics of the tool have sometimes been criticized (Pettinger 2005), with some experts stating that the results may not accurately identify personality type. However, many psychology and counseling professionals recommend the tool as a starting point for self-discovery about an individual's personality-based preferences and strengths, prompting further self-evaluation techniques.

When patients are challenged to clearly identify positive psychology interventions (PPIs) and activities that can be a good person-activity fit, medical practitioners might consider encouraging patients to explore insights about their preferences by taking the MBTI or a similar personality assessment online, reading the personality descriptions and reflecting on what aligns with their experiences. A sample abbreviated tool to be self-administered by patients is included below.

By becoming self-aware of personality-based preferences, individuals can prioritize PPIs that could be a good fit and potentially sustainable. Moreover, personality-based preferences can be used to guide the process of health behavior change and developing any healthy habit, including positive activities.

As with other recommendations that medical practitioners make, it's prudent to consider the culture of the individual. Although, the MBTI has been administered across countries and cultures, and has multicultural applications (Yoo & Robinson 2010), caution is advised. Some cultures may not be open to personality constructs. Moreover, people from different cultures might interpret the assessment questions differently or have cultural tendencies for certain personality types. The distribution of the personality types varies somewhat from country to country. But overall, the questionnaire, conducted across approximately 30 countries, has been found to be well-understood and applicable (Owens 2017).

Summary of Jungian Personality-Based Preferences

Each of us has a personality type with dominant preferences that can explain our patterns of gathering information from the world, interacting with it and making decisions. This personality framework based on constructs identified by Carl Jung is one approach to consider when prioritizing and personalizing PPIs. No single theory of personality and psychological makeup will be able to consistently explain and predict the activities that will be more engaging and sustainable for individuals. However, using a personality framework as a starting point and encouraging patients to make their own explorations with personality preferences as guidance can help hone down the positive activities. This personality framework is a lens for individuals to understand and leverage their personal strengths in order to boost self-confidence and positive experiences. Below is a brief explanation of the MBTI framework and an example of an abbreviated questionnaire.

References

Andrews A. Jung's Typology Revisited. *Jung J-Cult Psyche* 2014;8(4):92-98

Beebe J. Psychological types in Freud and Jung. *Jung J-Cult Psyche* 2013;6(3):58-71.

Lianov L. *My Happy Avatar: Use Your Mobile Device and Your Personality to Transform Your Health*, Fair Oaks, CA: HealthType, 2013.

Owens M. Is personality type universal across cultures? 2017, Feb. 28, www.truity.com [retrieved June 1, 2019].

Pettinger DJ. Cautionary comments regarding the Myers-Briggs Type Indicator. *Consul Psychol J Pract Res.* 2005;57(3):210-221.

Yoo JH, Robinson DH. Myers-Briggs Type Indicator (MBTI), multicultural applications. In Clauss-Ehlers CS (Eds.) *Encyclopedia of Cross-cultural School Psychology.* Boston, MA: Springer, 2010.

For Patients

Estimating Your Personality Preferences

You can estimate your Myers Briggs personality by doing one or more of the following:
- Review the lists of words and descriptors in the questionnaire below to estimate your personality.
- Take the MBTI questionnaire:
  - Long version that is computer-scored (accessible through a certified counselor; find more information at www.myersbriggs.org.)
  - Short version that you score (accessible from certified counselors)
  - Adapted versions, which may not be verified, are available online
  - Read detailed narrative descriptions of the type personalities, reflect and observe yourself to confirm the best fit. Many resources can be accessed online. Short descriptions of the most important aspects of the personalities are included below.

The following questionnaire is an abbreviated tool to help you:
- Think about which ways of thinking or behaving are most comfortable for you or you most prefer
- Prompt you to read further, do some self-reflection and talk to counseling professionals who have expertise in this personality framework.

Self-Rating Personality Questionnaire

- Select one option in each group.
- Even if you identify with both options, choose the one you tend to rely on most often or the one to which you are more strongly drawn.
- When you are in a situation that requires you to think or act quickly which would you likely think or do?

Source of Energy

Extraversion: Is drawn to and gets energy from the outer world and interacting with others
- Prefers to solve problems by talking to others
- Is in tune with the outside environment
- Is energized by being sociable and by having open discussions
- Has a variety of interests and prefers to know many people
- Reflects after speaking

OR

Introversion: Focuses on the inner world and gets energy from reflection and inward attention;
- Prefers to figure things out by inwardly reflecting
- Tends to be private and reveal only a few, selected things
- Has in-depth interests and prefers knowing a few people well
- Prefers to think before speaking
- Enjoys and is energized by spending time alone

What is your source of energy? Extraversion (E) or introversion (I)? _____

Gathering Information

Sensing: Focuses on gathering tangible information and notices details in the environment
- Is drawn to concrete facts
- Prefers practical, hands-on exercises to understand ideas
- Learns by doing step-by-step
- Prefers direct experience
- Focuses on the actual situation and the present reality

OR

iNtuition: Gathers information by seeing the big picture, sees connections between ideas, and notices patterns in the outer world
- Likes to consider future possibilities
- Prefers to figure out meanings behind patterns and information
- Focuses on ideas first before putting them into practice
- Trusts insights or hunches
- Needs to see the big picture and then learn the details and facts

How do you prefer to gather information? Sensing (S) or intuition (N)? _____

Decision Making

Thinking (T): Focuses on the logic when making a decision, is drawn to critique the situation, and identifies the pros/cons and the costs/benefits of options
- Tends to be analytical
- Seeks fairness by making sure everyone is treated equally
- Prefers to use objective criteria

- Looks at cause and effect
- Is usually swayed by logic

OR

Feeling (F): Focuses on what is important to self and others when making decisions; decides based on personal values

- Is energized by supporting others and making sure others feel appreciated
- First considers the impact of decisions on others
- Is drawn to harmonious situations and is uncomfortable with disagreements
- Places highest importance on personal values
- Is seen as compassionate and empathetic

How do you tend to make decisions? Thinking (T) or feeling (F)?_____

Arranging the Outer World

Judging (J): Prefers to have life planned and is drawn to come to closure on options

- Wants to have things decided and settled quickly
- Prefers that one project is completed before the next is begun

Likes to feel things are being done according to a pre-selected approach

- Prefers life to be organized and planned
- Is comfortable with routine

OR

Perceiving (P): Is drawn to flexibility, being spontaneous, and keeping things open-ended

- Likes to be open to make a change
- Is energized by last-minute pressure
- Easily adapts to change
- Enjoys multiple unfinished projects at the same time
- Is comfortable improvising

How do you prefer to have the outer world arranged? Judging (J) or Perceiving (P)?_____

What are the four options you selected? Write the four letters:_____

Find Your Main Personality Strength

ISTJ Introverted Sensing	ISFJ Introverted Sensing	INFJ Introverted Feeling	INTJ Introverted Feeling
ISTP Introverted Thinking	ISFP Introverted Feeling	INFP Introverted Feeling	INTP Introverted Thinking
ESTP Extraverted Sensing	ESFP Extraverted Sensing	ENFP Extraverted Intuition	ENTP Extraverted Intuition
ESTJ Extraverted Thinking	ESFJ Extraverted Feeling	ENFJ Extraverted Feeling	ENTJ Extraverted Thinking

Lianov L. *My Happy Avatar: Use Your Mobile Device and Presonality to Transform Your Health,* Fair Oaks, CA: HealthType, 2013.

How to Use Your Personality Strengths for Happiness and Health
Extraverted Sensing (ESFP, ESTP)

Those who prefer extraverted sensing are focused on the external, objective reality, factual and detailed perceptions. You likely seek out experiences that bring out the strongest sensations, especially enjoy beautiful surroundings, and are adept at fully experiencing the present moment. Examples of how this preference supports positive activities and healthy habits include:
- Meditating with full attention on breathing.
- Focusing on and enjoy the good physical sensations of exercise.

Introverted Sensing (ISFP, ISTJ)

If you prefer to gather information through introverted sensing, you tend to focus on internal impressions of what is happening in the external world. You rely on a wealth of internally stored memories/data and inward recollections of familiar experiences. Examples of how this preference supports positive activities and healthy habits include:
- Focusing on memories of how doing kind acts for others spurred good feelings and pride in yourself
- Recalling how running outside feels like childhood play

Extraverted Intuition (ENFP, ENTP)

If you prefer extraverted intuition, you tend to focus on possibilities, abstract observations and the pursuit of new ideas. You are likely interested in what is going on behind the scenes and see beyond what is in front of you. You are on the look-out for new opportunities, environments, activities, and possibilities. Examples of using this preference to support positive activities and healthy habits are:
- Brainstorming several ways to do a creative project
- Combining ideas from several exercise classes to create a new workout routine

Introverted Intuition (INFJ, INTJ)

If you prefer introverted intuition, you tend to focus on inspirations and insights without necessarily being able to give rational explanations for these insights. They are directed from within by "just knowing" possibilities and anticipating the future. Information may present itself to your awareness without external triggers. Examples of using this preference to support positive activities and healthy habit are:
- Developing a special way to express gratitude to someone based on an insight about that person
- Starting a new cooking routine based on insights about what healthy dishes would be easiest to make

Extraverted Thinking (ESTJ, ENTJ)

If you prefer the extraverted thinking preference, you are likely drawn to making objective decisions and value logical principles. You tend to put an order onto the outer world according to sets of principles. You might be more comfortable organizing, sorting, and applying criteria and logic than other personalities. Examples of using this preference to support positive activities and healthy habits are:
- Reaching out to expand your social network, because your read scientific studies about how social connections boost health
- Developing a process to keep a neighborhood walking group engaged

Introverted Thinking (ISTP, INTP)

If you prefer the introverted thinking preference, you tend to value objective decisions, but emphasize inwardly directed thinking to make those decisions. You likely enjoy spending time alone to consider your thoughts and ideas. You tend to be concerned with clarifying ideas logically and pursuing practical application of those ideas. You direct attention inward to figure out how to solve an obstacle, check for consistency of a plan and figure out how something works. Examples of using this preference to support positive activities and healthy habits are:
- Considering the science behind how different positive activities affect health and doing only those activities that align with your understanding of what works best
- Looking at the pros and cons of different physical activity routines to determine the best way of staying active

Extraverted Feeling (ESFJ, ENFJ)

If you prefer extraverted feeling, you tend to make decisions based on how others and personal relationships could be impacted. You likely seek to create harmonious conditions and strongly support social values. You give priority to arranging your external world according to what is importance in your social circle and responding to others' needs. Examples of using this process to support positive activities and healthy habits are:
- Getting input from family members on which positive activity could be made into a family activity (e.g. a family gratitude jar)
- Going out of your way to arrange an exercise schedule that works for a friend so that he can join you

Introverted Feeling (ISFP, INFP)

If you prefer introverted feeling, you tend to emphasize your values and people when making decisions, but you might keep your thoughts and feelings private. You tend to filter and evaluate situations through the lens of strong personal values. Examples of how to use this preference to positive activities and support healthy habits are:
- Volunteering at the animal shelter, because it supports your value to care for other creatures on earth
- Riding your bike to work, because it is better for the environment and for your health

Lianov L. *My Happy Avatar, Use Your Mobile Device and Personality to Transform Your Health*. Fair Oaks, California: HealthType, 2013.

Appendix F

Sample Positive Psychology Curriculum
Positive Psychology and Humanism in Medical Education

Designed by Carrie Barron at Dell Medical School and adapted for the American College of Lifestyle Medicine (ACLM)

Learning Objectives:
I. Master tenets of positive psychology skills, behaviors, practices and principles
II. Integrate strengths-based positive psychology interventions with traditional medical care
III. Identify personal character strengths for self-care, coping, professionalism and best practice

Method: Guided discussion, interactive exercises, short readings and reflection exercises in class

1) Introduction to Positive Psychology
   - Definition and evolution of positive psychology
   - Personal and professional uses of positive psychology practices
   - Strengths-based interventions and their impact on health
   - History: Abraham Maslow, Carl Rogers, Viktor Frankl and Martin Seligman researchers and humanist psychologists

   Literature: *Character Strengths and Virtues* by Martin Seligman and Chris Peterson excerpts

   Exercise: Each share something you love to do and why. Guided discussion on humanism, character, professionalism, identity, enlivening behaviors and how this connects to positive psychology

2) PERMA Optimal Living Template from Martin Seligman
   - PERMA: Positive Emotion, Engagement, Relationships, Meaning, Accomplishments
   - Philosophy, spirituality, science and religion research derived
   - Work. Love. Play. Quality Relationships: Core human needs across cultures and time
   - How can this be applied to interactions with patients? Especially if they are distressed?
   - Respect stress and explore realistic positives. "Best way out is always through." (Robert Frost, poet)

   Literature: *Flourish* by Martin Seligman, *Play* by Stuart Brown excerpts

   Exercise: Group: Guess what PERMA stands for. Partner and Discuss personal PERMA methods

3) Character Strengths for Good Work, Good Feeling and Clinical Acumen
   - Who we are, determines how we work. Authenticity and field alignment for flow.
   - Character traits and style: Hone and refine. Focus is not about deficits, but identification and ownership
   - Build character based on natural qualities. Greater/lesser strengths. Breeding via shared values
   - How can this be applied to clinical interactions?
   Literature: *Character Strengths and Virtues* by Seligman and Peterson excerpts
   Exercise: Virtues in Action Character Survey. Bring a story of how you used your character strengths

4) Relationships, Warm Exchanges and Coping through Human Connection
   - Relationships at work, best friends and intentional brief, warm interactions with colleagues
   - Mentors and role models with whom you can identify or who excite you
   - Intentional versus incidental positive interactions and a value system that celebrates warmth
   - Quality relationships for health and longevity. "Love at all levels of the organization" (Julia Abelson)
   - Interpersonal challenges. Interpersonal Medicine
   - Broaden and build theory; articles by Barbara Fredrickson
   Exercise: Write down 3 professional interactions that brought you positive emotion and your role in it. Populate an in-class list on the screen.

5) Gratitude/ Altruism and the Shadow Side of Self and Situations
   - Appreciative inquiry in work setting.
   - Research on volunteerism and sacrifice. Risks of being overly dutiful versus enlivened by giving
   - Compassion, meaning and connection are energizing and create neurophysiological changes
   - How can we help patients conjure gratitude if they feel defeated or down? Honoring and feeling
   the fear, disappointment and anger is path to the positive.
   - Layered listening as a form of generosity and addressing the shadow side
   Gratitude Works! by Robert Emmons excerpt. Articles on Positive Psychology 2.0 by Paul Wong and Barbara Held
   Exercise: What moved you, surprised you or cheered you this week? Positive Listening in pairs.
   Take home: Journaling before bed 3 good things that happened that day

6) Mindfulness and Minimalism
   - Slow medicine, reflection, mantras, meditation and personal ritual for creating calm
   - Change relationship to, thoughts about, response to stressor if you cannot change stressor
   - Efficiency of practice as a form of minimalism.
   - Mindfulness for patients or other calming, perspective-producing methods
   The Paradox of Choice by Barry Schwartz excerpt
   Exercise: Sit in silence for five minutes. Share personal forms of mindfulness.

7) Resilience, Moral Injury and Overcoming Obstacles
   - Cognitive shifts: Trading one thought for another or learning to conjure a more hopeful thought
   - More time versus control over time for well-being in medicine; moral injury issues
   - Meaning lifts moods (disaster research) and how we can apply to clinical work/joy in practice
   - Advocacy, assertion and expression of healthy anger and entitlement in systemic dysfunction
   - Rational and irrational self-criticism, triumphing over perfectionism, humiliation and shame
   Article on WOOP by Gabrielle Oettingen (woopmylife.org)
   Exercise: What is your WOOP (Wish. Outcome. Obstacle. Plan.)?

8) Self-Mastery and Grit
   - Autonomy, control, self-possession and self-discipline
   - Imagination, suppression and sticking to it as healthy defenses
   - Getting back on track and expecting falls
   Stanford Marshmallow Study on delayed gratification
   Grit by Angela Duckworth and *Mindset* by Carol Dweck excerpts
   Exercise: Discuss with a partner a time when you held back and waited, and it was worth it. Tell a story about working hard for something.

9) Happiness and Well-Being
   - Genetic set points and capacity for change
   - Practices that lead to true and lasting change
   - It is about a greater frequency of happy moments, not a permanent state
   - Immersion and everyday creativity (states of "flow") as actionable method for emotional well-being
   - How patients might use projects for health, both individual and community
   - "Show me a happy person and I will show you a project."
   The How of Happiness by Sonja Lyubomirsky excerpt
   Exercise: List projects that have been meaningful for you. Populate board and facilitate group discussion.

10) Flourishing
    - Customized approaches via self-knowledge
    - Positive psychology as sustenance
    - Well-being is a practice for ourselves and our patients. How do you choose, build and maintain well-being practices?
    - Owning what works and what does not. The "nos" are as important as the "yeses."
    - Self-possession, self-awareness and emotional intelligence as self-care
    Literature: *Flourish* by Martin Seligman excerpts
    Exercise: What is your well-being practice and how can you maintain it? What are some techniques for integrating meaningful and growth producing conversation into the clinical encounter? The aim is less about time, more about attunement. Group discussion.

Reading List Referenced in Curriculum

Duckworth, A. *Grit*. New York, NY: Scribner, 2018.

Dweck C. *Mindset*. New York, NY: Random House, 2006

Emmons R. *Gratitude Works!* San Francisco, CA: Jossey-Bass, 2013.

Lyubomirsky S. *The How of Happiness*. New York, NY: Penguin Books, 2007.

Schwartz, B. *The Paradox of Choice*. New York, NY: Eccopress, 2016.

Seligman ME, *Flourish*. New York, NY: Free Press, 2011

Seligman M, Peterson C. *Character Strengths and Virtues*. Washington DC: American Psychological Association/Oxford University Press, 2004.

About the Editor

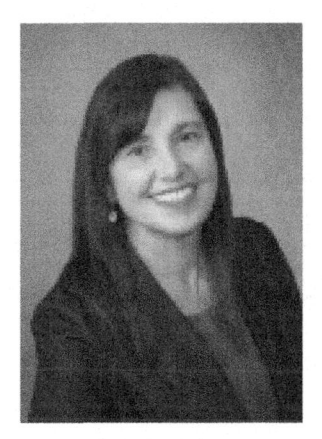

Liana Lianov, MD, MPH, FACLM, FACPM

As an innovative leader in lifestyle medicine, Dr. Lianov has advanced the field in the US and internationally and is pioneering its enhancement with the principles and science of positive psychology. She currently serves as Chair of the Happiness Science and Positive Health Committee of the American College of Lifestyle Medicine (ACLM), lead faculty for the ACLM Physician and Health Professional Well-Being Program, vice-chair of the American Board of Lifestyle Medicine, and President of the Positive Health and Wellness Division of the International Positive Psychology Association.

She led the development of the first of its kind intensive lifestyle medicine physician curriculum, sponsored by the American College of Preventive Medicine (ACPM) and ACLM, which set the stage for competency training in the field. The core competencies were developed by a national blue ribbon panel of health professional organizations, which she co-chaired, and were unveiled in her Journal of the American Medical Association benchmark article. For this program and related work, Dr. Lianov received the 2015 Distinguished Service Award from ACPM. Dr. Lianov is a past president of the ACLM, a past board regent of ACPM, and the former Healthy Lifestyles Division Director for the American Medical Association. She previously directed heart disease and stroke prevention, cancer detection, chronic diseases, and mental health services programs at the California Department of Health Services.

About the Authors

Grace Caroline Barron, MD is the Director of the Creativity and Resilience Program and Assistance Professor of Psychiatry at the University of Texas Austin, Dell Medical School. She is also a member of the American College of Lifestyle Medicine's Happiness Science and Positive Health Committee and served as lead liaison at Dell Medical School for the Inaugural Summit on Happiness Science in Health Care.

Kristen Collins, PhD has led a successful, long term career as a learning and development consultant at Wells Fargo and serves on the American College of Lifestyle Medicine's Happiness Science and Positive Health Committee. She was an International StrengthsFinder Scholar at Gallup Organization and earned her PhD in industrial-organizational psychology from Marshall Goldsmith School of Management, Alliant International University.

Ingrid Edshteyn, DO, MPH is a board certified lifestyle, preventive and obesity medicine physician in Los Angeles, California; she is the founder of Valia Lifestyle, a wellness studio that integrates these specialties into mind and body medicine. She also serves on the Happiness Science and Positive Health Committee of the American College of Lifestyle Medicine and has an executive masters in public health from Columbia University's Mailman School. Her vision is to embed positive mental well-being as the foundation of healthcare.

Janani Krishnaswami, MD, MPH is board certified in internal medicine and preventive medicine. She is a member of the American College of Lifestyle Medicine's Happiness Science and Positive Health Committee. Until recently, she served as the Program Director of the Preventive Medicine Residency Program at the University of Texas – Rio Grande Valley.

Rachel A. Millstein, PhD, MHS is a clinical health psychologist with a background in public health. She is an assistant professor and staff psychologist in the Behavioral Medicine Program and Cardiac Psychiatry Research Program at MGH and Harvard Medical School. Her research focuses on developing physical activity and diet interventions for chronic disease prevention.

Darren Morton, PhD is an internationally recognized lifestyle medicine expert and presenter, with special interest in the science of happiness. He has authored over fifty academic publications and four books, and has developed wellbeing programs that are used in over fifteen countries. He is certified by the International Board of Lifestyle Medicine and is a Fellow of the Australasian Society of Lifestyle Medicine.

Joe Raphael, DrPH, FACLM, MBA, MA, LMFT, CHES, HAPM is an integrative lifestyle medicine specialist, and has an MA in clinical psychology, an MBA in healthcare administration and a DrPH preventive care specialty. He is also a licensed marriage and family therapist, an American College of Lifestyle Medicine (ACLM) Fellow, a certified health education specialist, and a board-certified holistic alternative psychology master. He serves on the ACLM Happiness Science and Positive Health Committee and continues to work in advancing integrative lifestyle medicine, having successfully opened over 25 integrative medical practices.

Anne Wallace, PhD is Vice President of Applied Science at Beech Acres Parenting Center. Previously she served as a principal researcher at Humana and worked in Coaching Design and Development at Hummingbird Coaching Services. She is a member of the Happiness Science and Positive Health Committee at the American College of Lifestyle Medicine.